Clinical Governance
in Primary Care

Edited by

Tim van Zwanenberg

and

Jamie Harrison

Foreword by

Sir Michael Rawlins

Chairman, National Institute for Clinical Excellence

Radcliffe Medical Press Ltd
18 Marcham Road, Abingdon, Oxon OX14 1AA

British Library Cataloguing in Publication Data

A catalogue record for this book is available from the British Library.

ISBN 1 85775 396 8

Typeset by Advance Typesetting Ltd, Oxfordshire
Printed and bound by TJ International Ltd, Padstow, Cornwall

Contents

Foreword

Clinical governance is about trying to ensure that NHS patients get the best possible, and affordable, care. The range of activities encompassed in the term 'clinical governance' is, however, enormous and cannot be reduced to a mere checklist. For clinical governance is a philosophy: it seeks to equate the quality with the cost of care, and demands, from health professionals and health managers alike, personal responsibility for the totality of the experience that patients receive from the NHS.

This philosophy (or concept) is discomforting for those of us – whether in primary or secondary care – who already think that we do our best for patients under our care. It is difficult for any health professional to accept that we sometimes depart from 'best practice'. And it is only slightly less embarrassing when we discover that our own institutions, whether hospitals or general practices, have failed to provide the environment that patients can reasonably expect. Moreover, it is implicit that clinical governance and the commitment it demands can never be wholly satisfied. Yet it is in the striving, exponentially, for the goals that we seek that we are most likely to achieve them. For as we get close to utopia the goal posts will change, and more will be required of us.

Clinical Governance in Primary Care is a significant contribution to explaining, and exploring, clinical governance in all its manifestations. It offers a snapshot of the present and a vision for the future that I hope will enthuse and challenge all those involved in its implementation. It brings clinical governance alive and gives hope for the future.

Sir Michael Rawlins
Chairman, National Institute for Clinical Excellence
Professor of Clinical Pharmacology, University of Newcastle
September 1999

Preface

So what is clinical governance?

A man that looks on glass, on it may stay his eye; or if he pleaseth, through it pass, and then the heaven espy.

George Herbert

How comprehensive is our gaze? How willing are we to explore the world, and let it survey us? Even before the current power of globalisation, it had become clear to many that clinicians could no longer live in isolation, either from themselves, their colleagues or their clients (patients). The arrival of clinical governance is a public recognition of that fact.

The themes of clinical governance are those of quality, accountability, transparency and continuous improvement. It is said that such concerns can only flourish in a context of cooperation, teamwork and support. Much is made of the need to develop a 'no-blame' culture, yet ultimately someone or some group must take responsibility, and someone must lead.

In the light of such a discussion, many differing pictures of clinical governance have emerged, each with its own interest group. It is interesting to speculate on how to complete the sentence beginning 'Clinical governance is …'.

A window

The verse from George Herbert's hymn reminds us that to look upon a window offers us two choices. We can focus on the glass itself (near focus) or look beyond (distant focus). The near focus will hold us to a near, familiar view of our world – a limited horizon, where familiarity may breed complacency.

Better to look through the window, to gain the broader horizon and the challenge of the bigger picture. With that may come a glimpse of heaven, but equally an inkling of the road that must be travelled to get there. In this sense, clinical governance is the means by which organisations begin to see what their true objectives are.

A mirror

Windows also reflect light, as mirrors on the world. Some of the components of clinical governance can act like that, feeding back information, as they do, on what we are like, how we are doing. There are those who avoid the presence of mirrors.

Mirrors are valuable tools – ask any dentist, ENT surgeon, shaver or beautician. The reflections of the mirrors within clinical governance inform the thinking of teams and practitioners in the health service. They cannot, of course, ensure that any action is taken as a result. They are merely inert commentators, companions on the journey.

A system

System development, or systemisation, would be seen, by many, as the answer to difficulties in primary care. The problem is not, they would argue, the individuals concerned, but the context in which such individuals work together.

Certainly, teaching about how to initiate and develop systems in primary care has been slow for clinicians. Better management has, however, begun to rectify this. Clinical governance allows this process to accelerate, as the need for both good management systems and care pathways is highlighted.

A culture

To bring about cultural change is always difficult. Such change must be accompanied by a clearly articulated vision of what is envisaged, be realistic and well supported – financially and with human resources – and be seen as beneficial to all stakeholders. Otherwise, the change will only be superficial and cosmetic.

Clinical governance encourages a culture of excellence, partnership and accountability. As such, it must also find the resources to sustain its high ideals and maintain its vision across all the players in primary care.

An education

Some would wish to see clinical governance as purely an educational exercise. Clearly, the need for education about clinical governance, in addition to the clear role for continuing professional development within clinical governance itself, is self-evident.

Yet, there is a danger that the educational element could take over the whole agenda. It must see itself in partnership with the drive to better systems in primary care, and in the evolution of the culture of mutuality, trust and excellence which is already present in much of primary care.

A stained glass window

Returning to George Herbert, we may wish to finish with another type of window. A stained glass window comprises many, differently coloured, panes of glass, each set in place to form a coherent whole. Individually, each pane may be monochrome, uninspiring. Put all the panes together and a totally different effect emerges – a story told or an image expressed.

The ten components of clinical governance individually may not add up to much. Each is rather a building block, or coloured pane, in the construction of a larger and more significant work of art. Only when viewed in its entirety can such a work be judged. Lose one component and the story is incomplete, the image marred. Each component on its own is not enough.

Tim van Zwanenberg
Jamie Harrison
September 1999

List of contributors

Richard Baker	Director, Clinical Governance Research and Development Unit, Department of General Practice and Primary Health Care, University of Leicester
Arthur Bullough	Assistant Director, Primary Care Management, County Durham Health Authority
Liam Donaldson	Chief Medical Officer, Department of Health, London
Martin Eccles	Professor of Clinical Effectiveness, University of Newcastle
Christina Edwards	Regional Nurse Director, NHS Executive, Northern & Yorkshire
Ruth Etchells	Theologian and formerly Vice Chair, Durham FHSA and Chair of its Medical Services Committee
Janet Grant	Professor of Education in Medicine, Open University
Jeremy Grimshaw	Professor of Public Health, University of Aberdeen
Jamie Harrison	General Practitioner and GP Tutor, County Durham
Peter Hill	Postgraduate Dean, University of Newcastle
Robert Innes	Lecturer in Systematic Theology, St John's College, Durham
Mayur Lakhani	Lecturer, Clinical Governance Research and Development Unit, Department of General Practice and Primary Health Care, University of Leicester
Mike Pringle	Professor of General Practice, Nottingham University
Sir Michael Rawlins	Chairman, National Institute for Clinical Excellence
Marianne Rigge	Director, College of Health
John Spencer	Senior Lecturer in Primary Health Care, University of Newcastle
George Taylor	General Practitioner and Deputy Director of Postgraduate General Practice Education, University of Newcastle
Richard Thomson	Professor of Epidemiology and Public Health, University of Newcastle
Ian Watt	Professor of General Practice, York University
Tim van Zwanenberg	Professor of Postgraduate General Practice, University of Newcastle

About this book

Who is it for?

We hope everyone involved in primary care will find useful information in this book. Clinical governance is after all 'everybody's business'. Primarily we have aimed to meet the needs of those charged with leading the development of clinical governance at the level of primary care group, primary care team, community health service or primary care trust, and health authority. The contents should be of interest and relevance to all professional groups, although we recognise that much of the material is drawn from general practice and community nursing with less reference to the other allied professions. For simplicity we have used the term *primary care group* throughout, recognising that this is the organisational arrangement in England. There are equivalent primary care organisations, with different names, in the other parts of the United Kingdom. The issue of clinical governance is generic to them all.

What does it contain?

The book is intended to provide a description of the principles of clinical governance in primary care, and practical information about many of its component processes. In general, definitions, evidence and practical experience have been emphasised. Many of the chapters point to other sources of information. We have made no attempt at a detailed description of the supporting structures and processes which are being developed on a national basis to support clinical governance – in England, the National Institute for Clinical Excellence and the Commission for Health Improvement, and National Service Frameworks. Moreover, we have tried to provide information that might be useful to primary care staff in implementing, for example, national guidelines.

How to use it?

The book is divided into three parts. The first (Chapters 1 and 2) sets the scene. The conceptual and political origins of clinical governance are traced, and the significance of organisational culture is emphasised. Stress is placed on the importance of patients, people and processes. The second part (Chapters 3–13) is arranged around four domains of clinical governance – humane care, clinical effectiveness, risk management, and personal and professional development. It describes a range of practical processes that support the development of clinical governance. The third part (Chapters 14–16) looks ahead, offering a critique of how professionalism might develop in the future against a background of increasing expectation.

Readers will have different interests and can use the book accordingly.

- You may wish to read the book from page 1 to the end.
- You have a specific interest in clinical audit (Chapters 5 and 6) or complaints (Chapter 10).
- You need to understand the pressure for accountability in the NHS (Chapters 1, 3 and 15).
- You want to consider the implications for education and training (Chapters 12–14).
- You keep hearing about 'poor performance' and want to know more (Chapters 1 and 11).

Periodically, as clinical governance develops, primary care organisations will wish to review their progress and plan future development. One such assessment by a primary care team, using the chapter headings of the book, is shown on pages xii–xiii. Frameworks for these assessments have also been produced by the Department of Health,[1] by the Royal College of General Practitioners,[2] and by Richard Baker and his colleagues.[3]

References

1 Department of Health (1999) *Clinical Governance: quality in the new NHS*. Health Service Circular: HSC(99)065. Department of Health, London.

2 Royal College of General Practitioners (1999) *Clinical Governance: practical advice for primary care in England and Wales*. RCGP, London.

3 Baker R, Lakhani M, Fraser R and Cheater F (1999) A model for clinical governance in primary care groups. *BMJ*. **318**: 779–83.

Baseline assessment by a primary care team

Process	Existing activity	Planned activity
Evidence-based practice	• Some team members use internet • Two doctors appraise guidelines • Guideline folder in preparation • PRODIGY installed	• More systematic filtering of guidelines • Complete guideline folder • Explore development of computer system support
Disseminating good practice	• Team members occasionally circulate information from journals, courses • Regular programme of continuing professional development (CPD)	• Encourage more circulation of information tit-bits
Quality improvement processes	• Audits are undertaken fairly regularly	• Systematic annual audit programme, e.g. diabetes in May, heart disease in June, etc.
Appropriate use of data	• Annual activity analysis • Audit of disease management • Analysis of prescribing	• None specific
Reducing clinical risk	• Acknowledged lack of knowledge, activity and expertise	• Devote next time-out to risk analysis, involving whole team
Significant event analysis	• Occasional formal significant event analysis meeting • Supportive team encourages 'debriefing' after near misses, etc.	• Continue occasional formal meetings • Develop other opportunities for debriefing on informal basis
Lessons from complaints	• Only one written complaint in last two years	• Routine sharing of information about any complaint received

	• Lessons from complaints *not* shared • Not yet culture which welcomes complaints, although informal feedback between team members is good • Exploration of patient involvement in progress	• Continue to explore methods of patient involvement with view to testing among specific groups, e.g. people with diabetes
Poor performance tackled	• Feedback among team members is the norm	• None specific
Continuing professional development (CPD)	• Programme of weekly lunch-time multidisciplinary CPD meetings • Programme of receptionist training • Doctors have engaged in peer appraisal – with planned follow-up • Attached staff are beginning to develop personal development plans (PDPs)	• Need to bring personal development plans together in Practice Professional Development Plan (PPDP) • Develop peer appraisal further
Leadership development	• Roles of executive partner and practice manager well established and effective • Role of nursing representative at weekly management meetings established • Team has good sense of direction from previous time-outs set out in practice development plan	• New development plan needs to be completed • Triumvirate of executive partner, practice manager and nursing representative to lead on clinical governance – identifying themselves to primary care group

Based on a rapid appraisal by the primary care team at Collingwood Surgery, North Shields.

Acknowledgements

We are grateful for the support and help of a wide variety of people in producing this book. In particular, we would like to thank all the contributors for their enthusiasm and hard work. Many colleagues have helped clarify our thinking by asking questions and making comments on presentations we have given on the subject in various parts of the country. The primary care group clinical governance leads in our region have allowed us to participate in their small group discussions, from which we have learned much about their early concerns and challenges. Stuart Warrender gave us the idea that clinical governance is like a stained glass window. Murray Lough's paper on clinical governance in primary care in Scotland stimulated us to think about the domains of clinical governance. Laura Stroud, Chair of North Tyneside Community Health Council, helped us understand the patients' view. Christina Edwards advised us on nursing matters. Tony Jameson from the North-East Change Centre facilitated a discussion on the future of professionalism with a group of senior managers from health and social services, clinicians, theologians, patients' representatives and politicians. We thank them all for their thoughtful ideas and comments. David Thorne and Pfizer have kindly supported a number of workshops and meetings we have organised. We have, as ever, relied on our primary care team colleagues at Collingwood Surgery, North Shields, and Cheveley Park Medical Centre, Durham. They have given us not only examples of good practice, but also constant reminders of reality. We thank our partners for their support, and their forbearance at dining rooms submerged in papers. Heidi Allen from Radcliffe Medical Press has encouraged us throughout. Beverly Brennan and Claire Goodwin have helped Angela McLaughlin, who has worked efficiently and with great calm and good humour, to produce the final typescript. Our considerable thanks are due to them.

To our children
Saffron and Luke van Zwanenberg
and
Sarah, Timothy and Nicola Harrison

Clinical governance is a system through which NHS organisations are accountable for continuously improving the quality of their services and safeguarding high standards of care by creating an environment in which excellence in clinical care will flourish.

Gabriel Scally and Liam Donaldson

Clinical governance is a framework for the improvement of patient care through commitment to high standards, reflective practice, risk management, and personal and team development.

Royal College of General Practitioners

Primary care is first contact, continuous, comprehensive and co-ordinated care provided to individuals and populations undifferentiated by age, gender, disease or organ system.

Barbara Starfield

PART 1

Setting the scene

CHAPTER ONE

Clinical governance: a quality concept

Liam Donaldson

If you always do what you always did, you always get what you always got.

Granny Donaldson

> This chapter defines clinical governance and describes its origins. The importance of organisational culture in the new primary care groups and trusts is emphasised. Clinical governance involves learning from both good and poor clinical practice.

Introduction

Clinical governance was one of the central ideas in a range of proposals to modernise the National Health Service[1] (NHS) contained in a White Paper produced by the incoming Labour government in the late 1990s.

From the post-war years at the beginning of the NHS, through the 1960s, to the periods of cost containment in the 1970s and 1980s, and into the era of health system reform of the early 1990s, concepts and methods of quality in healthcare underwent a quiet revolution.

In the early years of the NHS, quality was implied, assured by the training, skill and professional ethos of its staff. Standards of care were undoubtedly high for their time and the nationalisation of health services and facilities brought about by the creation of the NHS undoubtedly improved many past inequalities in access and provision. However, quality was essentially viewed through paternalistic eyes with the patient a passive recipient of care. The 1960s saw a growth in thinking about concepts of quality, much of it emanating from North America, notably Donabedian's quality triad (structures, processes, outcomes)[2] which has endured over more than 30 years. Despite these more sophisticated notions of quality emanating from academics and health service researchers the vision was seldom realised in practice.

By the 1980s, management was beginning to become established within the health systems of many parts of the world. In the NHS, accountability for the performance of a health organisation came as career general managers replaced health service administrators.[3] Initially resented by many professional staff, management gradually extended to the running of clinical services with the creation of clinical directorates and budgets.

The desire to build on these trends led, in the late 1980s and early 1990s, to attempts to design incentives for efficiency and quality into the NHS system itself. The resulting internal market for public healthcare in Britain split responsibility for the purchasing and provision of healthcare between health authorities and general practice fundholders (they were allocated budgets to purchase) and NHS trusts (they competed to provide services and gained a share of these budgets).[4] The theory was that the internal market would simulate the behaviour of a real market and drive up quality whilst reducing costs. This concept of quality improvement remained controversial and many professional staff working within the NHS were not confident that it could or did work.

The 1997 White Paper[1] signalled the dismantling of the internal market and its replacement with a system based on partnership and collaboration, not competition. With it came a new duty of quality which was placed on all health organisations in the NHS, embodied at a local level by a responsibility to develop clinical governance.

Throughout this period of evolution of health service policy in relation to quality, initiatives by professional bodies in Britain continued to advance standards of practice. However, in the past these have not always taken shape at a local level so that practical approaches to quality improvement are developed in an integrated fashion.

Organisations and people

Clinical governance is essentially an organisational concept. This is made clear by the way in which it was first defined: 'a framework through which NHS organisations are accountable for continuously improving the quality of their services and safeguarding high standards of care by creating an environment in which excellence in clinical care will flourish.'[5]

The elements of accountability, of ensuring that positive outcomes are delivered and of creating the right environment for good practice to flourish are all organisational features.

Organisational culture, what it constitutes, what determines whether it is beneficial and how to change it, has not, on the whole, been studied systematically in the healthcare field, although it features extensively in the management sciences research literature.[6] However, there are a number of generic features which many health service managers and professionals would recognise from their good and bad experiences during the progression of their careers (Table 1.1). Yet, achieving the right culture is seen as the most

Table 1.1   Ten key features of a positive culture within a health organisation

- Good leadership at all levels
- Open and participative style
- Good internal communication
- Education and research valued
- Patient and user focus
- Feedback on performance routine
- Good use of information
- Systematic learning from good practice and failure
- External partnerships strong
- Produces leaders of other health organisations

important element in implementing the clinical governance programme within the NHS.[7]

Much of the past work on improving quality through organisational development within the NHS has been directed at hospital or community health services rather than primary care. Whilst a general practice, with its extended primary care team, was certainly an organisation, it was small in scale; the framework of accountability was diffuse and devolved, and the element of management was firmly in support of clinical activities rather than leading and placing responsibilities on the health professionals within the practice.

The creation of primary care groups and trusts, which began in April 1999,[8] changes all this. Primary care groups, 481 in England serving average populations of 100 000 and containing as many as 50 general practitioners (GPs), are entirely new entities. They will have boards and chief executives. Moreover, primary care groups which have opted to become primary care trusts inherit staff formerly employed by NHS trusts (either 'community', 'mental health and community' or integrated 'acute and community'). The decoupling of these groups of community health staff from the pre-existing NHS trusts adds further to the composition of the new primary care bodies.

The new primary care structures are thus substantial new organisations, which will, over time, create their own cultures. Individual GPs and other health professionals will become committed to success at the corporate level, as well as at the level of their own clinical teams. In setting out the agenda for the new NHS, and in particular the primary care organisations, the government has described it as a long-term agenda of development.[8]

Well into the 21st century, primary care groups and trusts will be developing as organisations leaving behind the small-practice ethos of the early years of the NHS. This organisational development task will be a challenge in itself but building into the new organisations a working model of clinical governance will be an essential early task. The first stages of implementation of clinical governance involve four key steps[7]:

- establish leadership, accountability and working arrangements
- carry out a baseline assessment of capacity and capability

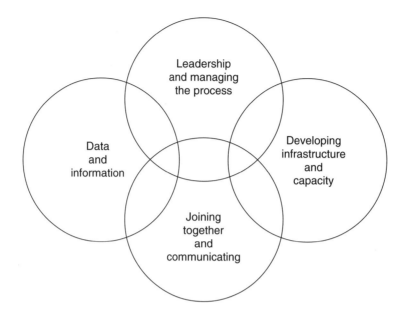

Figure 1.1   Developing clinical governance: leading change.

- formulate and agree a development plan in the light of this assessment
- clarify reporting arrangements for clinical governance within board and annual reports.

The precise approach to implementation is a matter for local discretion, but it seems particularly likely that the lead clinician responsible for clinical governance within the new primary care organisations will want to establish a team probably drawn together on a multidisciplinary basis.

One possible model (Figure 1.1) would see different members of the team taking responsibility for key functions, such as ensuring that different aspects of the quality improvement programme are 'joined together', that the important information and information technology needs of the programme are being met, that an overview of progress is taken and that communication is good.

Whatever the leadership arrangements, essential elements are that the whole organisation is involved in a way that promotes inclusivity and that there is clear leadership and communication from the top (Table 1.2).

A thorough analysis of the organisation's services from a quality perspective to identify their strengths and weaknesses establishes the baseline from which a development plan can be drawn up.

In closing the gap between the current position and the desired future state of improved quality a number of questions need to be addressed (Table 1.3).

There is little doubt that the development of primary care groups and trusts as cohesive organisations, with clear corporate goals and objectives directed towards quality

Table 1.2 Clinical governance: key elements of leadership arrangements

- **Inclusivity**, ensuring that all key groups in the organisation are involved and kept fully informed about the purpose and progress of the clinical governance programme.
- **Commitment from the top,** reporting and having free access to the chief executive and the board, particularly when problems need to be resolved or barriers to progress have been identified.
- **Good external relationships**, forging strong, open, working partnerships with health organisations and other agencies in the locality.
- **Constancy of purpose**, keeping the programme on course and not being deflected from the goals that the organisation has set itself.
- **Accounting for progress**, being able at all times to provide a comprehensive overview of progress with the clinical governance programme throughout the organisation.
- **Communicating**, to all staff in the organisation and to external partners on a regular basis.

Source: Department of Health.[7]

Table 1.3 Closing the quality gap in a service: some important questions

- Is the solution a workforce one (more staff, different skills)?
- Is the solution an education and training one (development of existing staff)?
- Is the solution a realignment with patients' perspectives on quality (greater involvement of service users and carers in planning the improvements)?
- Is the solution an infrastructure one (new facilities or equipment)?
- Is the solution to remedy information deficits (better information, information technology, access to both)?
- Is the solution substantial investment of new resources (prioritisation through the local Health Improvement Programme)?

improvement and the development of their staff, will be the keys to the success of clinical governance in primary care.

Shifting the quality curve

A simple composite measure of quality, if one existed, would see healthcare organisations distributed along a curve (Figure 1.2) – the worst performers at the left-hand tail, the leading edge organisations at the right. The greatest impact on quality, i.e. the biggest move of the curve towards the right, will be achieved by shifting the mean. In other words, helping organisations whose performance is average (or just above or just below average) to achieve the levels of the best. However, the two tails of the distribution cannot be ignored. Poor organisational performance and serious service failure are phenomena which are probably uncommon in relation to the totality of healthcare provided in the NHS. So eliminating them would not cause the quality curve to shift a great deal overall. Nevertheless, such events have very serious, sometimes catastrophic, repercussions for individual patients and their families. Specific incidents are often portrayed by the media as if they were the tip of an iceberg of similar problems within health services. So their

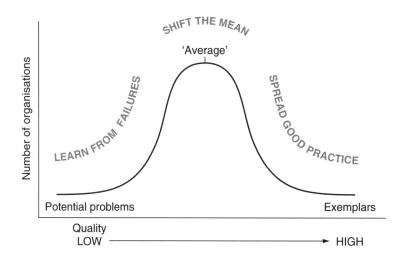

Figure 1.2   Variation in the quality of organisations.

occurrence, and the media criticism which attends them, can damage public confidence in services.

Relatively little research has been conducted to explore reasons why health organisations fail. Experience suggests that organisations which are poorly led, which are defensive to criticism, where there is no ethos of teamwork and where there are weak management systems will be those that are prone to failure.[10] Greater understanding of error in medicine is likely to show that it is a mixture of individual and organisational problems that lead to serious failures in standards of care.[11,12]

Finding ways to learn lessons from service failure within primary care groups and trusts will be one important part of clinical governance. It will be another manifestation of the new primary care services becoming effective organisations.

The activities of sharing and adopting good practice concentrate attention on the right-hand tail of the quality curve in Figure 1.2. To do so will help to shift the overall curve to the right but there are other reasons for concentrating on good practice. First, it is not something which the NHS has been good at in the past. So, patients in one part of the country will have benefited from an innovation in service delivery whilst those elsewhere will have been denied its benefit. This is surely inequitable. Second, sharing good practice encourages a learning approach to service development and is likely to have other quality spin-offs in the kind of culture it creates. Third, an increasing amount of clinical decision-making will be based upon following good practice guidelines so a similar ethos needs to be developed in service organisation and delivery – recognising models of service which can be transferred to other services to create improved quality.

The emergence of the evidence-based medicine movement, which started in Canada[13] and rapidly became international in its scope, has encouraged the adoption of more rigour in clinical decision-making. Numerous examples[14] exist of research evidence having been slow (or failed entirely) to enter routine practice so that sub-optimal care is delivered to patients. The philosophy of evidence-based medicine has been the impetus to the standards-based approach to quality, as exemplified in the NHS by the establishment in 1999 of the National Institute for Clinical Excellence (NICE). Addressing these issues in primary care groups and trusts is not perhaps as straightforward as it is in specialist areas of hospital medicine. This is partly because of the degree of uncertainty in many patient encounters in primary care and the absence of a diagnostic label upon which there is a strong body of research evidence on clinical effectiveness. Nevertheless, promoting an evidence-based culture will mean ensuring that all health professionals have been trained in the critical appraisal of research evidence. It will mean having available and knowing how to access specialist information resources (such as that provided by the Cochrane Collaboration[15]). It will mean ensuring that health professionals in primary care are able to use evidence in the interest of clinical audit and other quality improvement methodologies.

Less experience has been gained in evaluating service models than clinical interventions. A 'good' service (say) for diabetic people will often gain its reputation by being valued by patients and referring practitioners rather than by formal evaluation. If the NHS is to ensure that good practice is replicated then ways will have to be found of identifying the organisational ingredients that amount to success.

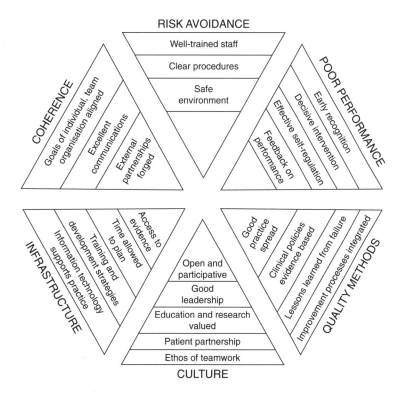

Figure 1.3　　Integrating approaches of clinical governance.

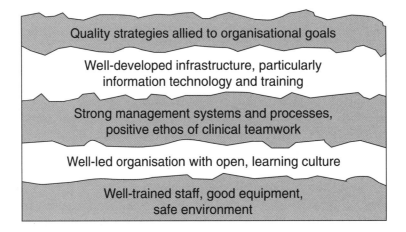

Figure 1.4   Clinical governance: drilling to the core.

Undertaking clinical governance thus involves learning from experience of both good and bad practice. It involves addressing the diverse aspects of quality improvement which are carried out to some extent in all organisations, but ensuring that they are performed well and systematically everywhere and carried out within an integrated quality strategy (Figure 1.3). Drilling to the core of a primary care group or trust which is well governed clinically will show the organisational layers built up from environment to infrastructure to organisational goals (Figure 1.4).

Addressing poor clinical performance

In the early 1990s, the NHS was dogged by a series of newspaper headlines about adverse outcomes of care arising from apparently poor clinical performance by individual doctors. Two episodes in particular created a major watershed in public and professional attitudes to this problem. The events that occurred in the children's heart surgery service at the Bristol Royal Infirmary,[16] which led to three doctors being struck off the Medical Register after the longest hearing in the General Medical Council's (GMC) history, and the case of Mr Rodney Ledward, a gynaecologist in Kent who was also struck off by the GMC following allegations about his standards of practice which attracted lurid headlines.[17] Both incidents are the subject of inquiries ordered by the Secretary of State for Health.

By the late 1990s it was clear that the public no longer had confidence in the mixture of professional self-regulation and NHS disciplinary procedures that had been the basis of dealing with poor clinical performance since the NHS began. There were enough examples of serious problems with competence and conduct, which had apparently been known about on informal networks for some time with no action being taken until matters reached crisis point. There were too many examples of lengthy suspensions of doctors which often cost the taxpayer large sums of money as legal wrangling ensued. There were other examples of doctors who had caused serious problems in one place, being allowed to move on and practise elsewhere without patients being aware that there were concerns about their practice.

Poor clinical performance is a complex issue.[18] It can present in a wide variety of ways, for example: failure to recognise, diagnose and treat illness adequately; poor attitude and disruptive behaviour; high levels of complications in patients treated; poor record keeping; and disorganised practice. A proportion of poorly performing doctors will have ill-health or addiction problems which may not be recognised until a patient suffers harm.

Most experience of poor clinical performance in the NHS has been gained in dealing with hospital doctors who pose such difficulties. Poorly performing GPs, because of their independent contractor status, and because their practice is by nature less subject to day-to-day observation by other members of a clinical team, have been recognised less often than perhaps they should have been. Although there have been serious cases dealt with by the GMC, they probably do not reflect the true extent of the problem. The proposed extension of the GMC's powers to determine every five years whether a doctor is fit to continue in practice, so-called revalidation,[19] the broadened concept of the duties of a doctor as set down by the GMC,[20] and the advent of clinical governance itself will have a profound effect on individual GPs and on the functioning of primary care groups and trusts within which they work.

As will be the case for other NHS organisations, the new primary care structures are expected through clinical governance to create the kind of organisation in which many of the problems of poor professional practice seen in the past will be prevented. This will mean creating strong programmes of continuing professional development, designing systems to monitor and detect poor outcomes of care early, and to intervene where poor practice is the cause. It will mean, over time, developing effective appraisal systems for all staff.

For the individual practitioner it will mean keeping up-to-date, participating in the clinical governance programme of the primary care group or trust to the full, and recognising problems with his or her own performance and seeking help. Importantly, it will no longer be acceptable professional behaviour to fail to draw attention to concerns about serious problems with a colleague's standard of practice.

Conclusions

Clinical governance is a powerful, new and comprehensive mechanism for ensuring that high standards of clinical care are maintained throughout the NHS and that the quality of services is continuously improved. Primary care services are at the centre of a programme to modernise the NHS introduced by the Labour government, which came to power in the spring of 1997. The new primary care structures which have been created, must develop as organisations with all that entails for their constituent practices and practitioners. There will need to be a commitment to corporate goals and strategies, the creation of leadership and accountability arrangements and above all the establishment of the right kind of culture. Clinical governance must be woven into the fabric of the new organisations from the outset.

The prize to be gained is enormous as the benefit of improved quality flows to patients up and down the country. Important tests of the success of the new arrangements will be their ability to prevent the kinds of serious service failures which hit the headlines during the early 1990s, and to recognise early and resolve cases of poor clinical performance before they result in disaster.

Practical points

- Initiatives aimed at improving quality in the past have not been integrated.
- Clinical governance is a new and comprehensive mechanism.
- All health organisations in the NHS now have a duty of quality.
- Achieving the right organisational culture in primary care groups and trusts will be critical to success.
- The first stages of implementation involve four key steps – leadership arrangements, baseline assessment, formulation of a plan and arrangements for monitoring.
- The aim of clinical governance is to 'shift the quality curve' to the right.
- Finding ways to learn from service failure in primary care is one important element.
- Learning from and reproducing good practice is also crucial.
- Many of the problems of poor professional practice should be prevented through clinical governance.
- Clinical governance must be 'woven into the fabric' of the new primary care organisations from the start.

References

1   Department of Health (1997) *The New NHS: modern, dependable*. Cm 3807. The Stationery Office, London.

2   Donabedian A (1966) Evaluating the quality of medical care. *Milbank Memorial Fund Quarterly*. **4**: 166–206.

3   Griffiths R (1983) *NHS Management Enquiry*. Department of Health and Social Security, London.

4   Department of Health (1989) *Working for Patients*. Cm 555. The Stationery Office, London.

5   Department of Health (1998) *A First Class Service: quality in the new NHS*. Health Service Circular: HSC(98)113. Department of Health, London.

6   Hastings C (1993) *The New Organization: growing the culture of organizational networking*. McGraw-Hill, London.

7   Department of Health (1999) *Clinical Governance: quality in the new NHS*. Health Service Circular: HSC(99)065. Department of Health, London.

8   Department of Health (1998) *The New NHS: modern and dependable primary care groups delivering the agenda*. Health Service Circular: HSC(98)228. Department of Health, London.

9   Scally G and Donaldson LJ (1998) Clinical governance and the drive for quality improvement in the new NHS in England. *BMJ*. **317**: 61–5.

10 Donaldson LJ and Gray JAM (1988) Clinical governance: a quality duty for health organisations. *Quality in Health Care*. **7**(Suppl 1): S37–S44.

11 Leape L (1977) A systems analysis approach in medical error. *Journal of Evaluation in Clinical Practice*. **3**: 213–22.

12 Donaldson LJ (1999) Medical mishaps: a managerial perspective. In: MM Rosenthal, L Mulcahy and S Lloyd-Bostock (eds) *Medical Mishaps: pieces of the puzzle*. Open University Press, Buckingham.

13 Evidence-based Medicine Working Group (1992) Evidence-based medicine: a new approach to teaching the practice of medicine. *JAMA*. **268**: 2420–5.

14 Donaldson LJ (1996) Impact of management on outcomes. In: M Peckham and R Smith (eds) *Scientific Basis of Health Services*. BMJ Books, London.

15 The Cochrane Library (1998) *The Cochrane Collaboration*, Issue 5. Update Software, Oxford.

16 Smith R (1998) Regulation of doctors and the Bristol inquiry. Both need to be credible to both the public and doctors. *BMJ*. **317**: 1539–40.

17 Dyer C (1998) Obstetrician accused of committing a series of surgical blunders. *BMJ*. **317**: 767.

18 Donaldson LJ (1994) Doctors with problems in an NHS workforce. *BMJ*. **308**: 1277–82.

19 Irvine D (1999) The performance of doctors: the new professionalism. *Lancet*. **353**: 1174–7.

20 General Medical Council (1995) *Good Medical Practice*. GMC, London.

CHAPTER TWO

Clinical governance in primary care

Tim van Zwanenberg and Christina Edwards

The good of the people is the chief law

Cicero

This chapter describes how clinical governance involves a coherent range of processes, which together assure the quality of clinical care. The involvement of patients from the start, and the support and development of primary care staff are important aspects of clinical governance in primary care.

In recent years primary care has moved to take up an increasingly pivotal position in the NHS, such that the newly formed primary care groups and their successor trusts are responsible not only for managing primary care, but also for commissioning much of secondary care, and for improving the public health.[1] Against this background of increased power, influence and responsibility, accountability for the quality of primary care has inevitably assumed greater importance. Primary care groups and trusts are now to be responsible for the clinical governance of primary care – giving patients, healthcare professionals, managers and government assurances about the *goodness* of clinical care provided.

The pressure for this level of accountability arises, in part, from the public interest in recent celebrated cases of malpractice. But even amidst the furore after the Bristol case cautionary voices sounded. Richard Smith, editor of the *British Medical Journal*, observed that if the case led 'to an environment where we concentrate on removing bad apples rather than on improving the whole system, then both patients and doctors will suffer'.[2] And Professor David Hunter pointed out that 'dependence on trust in the medical profession may not be fashionable in an age of consumerism, but that does not lessen its validity'.[3] Both were commenting specifically on doctors, but the same principles apply to all health professionals. Mechanisms are needed which help to develop all, and which guarantee trust.

There are two further reasons for the heightened interest in the quality assurance of primary care. First, there are evident variations in the range of services provided and in the quality of those services.[4] The very nature of primary care and the way it is organised in the UK has encouraged diversity, and over the years this has stimulated and promoted much innovation. At its extreme, however, this diversity has led to unacceptable differences between the good and the poor.

Second, these inconsistencies have never been fully remedied by the many attempts at quality improvement. Too often, initiatives like the development of clinical audit have been taken up by only the 'leading edge' primary care teams. And in general, programmes of development have been isolated one from another. This has resulted in fragmentation,[5] and a good deal of frustration among progressive primary care professionals and managers.

Nevertheless these initiatives, particularly the work of the professional bodies and the medical audit advisory groups (MAAGs) and their successors, have prepared the ground well. And in a historical context it has been argued that MAAGs, for example, should be seen as part of the expanding culture of greater objectivity and critical analysis that has burgeoned in clinical practice over the last two decades.[6] Although MAAGs were intended to concentrate on medical audit, they have steadily and appropriately embraced multiprofessional clinical audit and the wider aspects of quality development in primary care practice.

Clinical governance in primary care

Clinical governance then, offers a coherent framework for bringing together the disparate strands of quality improvement. The original government White Paper, *The New NHS: modern, dependable*, identified ten component processes of clinical governance, and proposed that a 'quality organisation' will ensure that they are in place.[7] Each of these processes is the subject of a chapter in this book.

They have been called 'the ten commandments of clinical governance' (*see* Box 2.1), but in truth there could have been only eight or nine (a number of the components overlap) or 11 or more (some important components are not listed). The significant point is that each on its own will not suffice. The processes, some of which are quite narrow whereas others are more broad, need to be linked so that clinical governance becomes 'a systematic set of mechanisms',[8] which provides primary care organisations with the right balance of accountability and continuous quality improvement.[9] Most of the activities involved in clinical governance are already happening, more or less – some

---

Box 2.1:   The 'ten commandments of clinical governance'

1   Evidence-based practice with the infrastructure to support it (*see* Chapter 4).
2   Good practice, ideas and innovations systematically disseminated (*see* Chapter 5).
3   Quality improvement processes, for example clinical audit (*see* Chapter 6).
4   High-quality data to monitor clinical care (*see* Chapter 7).
5   Clinical risk reduction programmes (*see* Chapter 8).
6   Adverse events detected and openly investigated; and the lessons learned promptly applied (*see* Chapter 9).
7   Lessons for clinical practice systematically learned from complaints made by patients (*see* Chapter 10).
8   Problems of poor clinical performance recognised at an early stage and dealt with (*see* Chapter 11).
9   All professional development programmes reflect principles of clinical governance (*see* Chapter 12).
10 Leadership skill development at clinical team level (*see* Chapter 13).

---

more, some less. The big idea is to promote and marshal all the activities to develop the organisation as a whole.

The outcome of an early workshop on clinical governance, involving patient representatives, primary care practitioners and health service managers, is pertinent here.[10] The participants concluded that the arrangements for clinical governance in primary care would have to meet a number of paramount needs:

- the need to secure public confidence – including the involvement of patients and carers from the start
- the need to be inclusive of all practitioners
- the need to support the continuous improvement of the many (who are trying to do their best)
- the need to map and make use of existing activities and resources
- the need to provide an explicit and effective process for dealing with unacceptable practice.

At each level of primary care, individual, practice, primary care team, primary care group or trust, success will depend on the interaction of three key parts of the system – patients, people, i.e. staff, and processes (*see* Box 2.2).

Patients

Although there has been much rhetoric about the involvement of patients in planning service development and in enhancing the quality of care, and there are plenty of examples of effective good practice, effective involvement is by no means universal. Much

---

Box 2.2:   The three key contributors to clinical governance in primary care

Patients
- want to contribute
- should be involved early on
- hold the NHS in high regard

People
- make primary care work
- need support
- must demonstrate fitness to practise

Processes
- the 'ten commandments of clinical governance'
- external accreditation
- protection of patient information

---

of the experience, in general practice at least, has been focused on studies of patient satisfaction, yet responding to a questionnaire is hardly engagement. Practice-based patient participation groups have been tried, but are perceived by many as being the preserve at best of the middle classes, and at worst of special interest groups or lobbies.

Yet the argument for involvement seems irrefutable. There is a need to 'move to an active rather than passive trust between doctors and patients, where doctors share uncertainty'.[2] For so long as the health service sustains a paternalistic attitude, so patients will respond like children and not help with negotiating the inevitable trade-offs in everyday practice. Here is what the patients' representative, the chair of a Community Health Council, said at the workshop.[10]

I am very pleased to be here today because I believe that it is important to involve all the stakeholders in such an important debate right from the start. It is more usual for patients to be involved at a later stage, when the agenda has been set and all we can do is react to it. In my view a much more satisfactory set of outcomes is likely with full and equal partnerships from the beginning.

But you shouldn't just involve patients because the government says you have to. There are plenty of other good reasons why patients should be involved. For example:

- *evidence-based practice is no good if patients don't comply with it;*
- *patients are becoming better informed and practitioners need to re-evaluate the doctor–patient relationship in the light of this; and*
- *patient involvement may result in a better set of performance measures that more realistically reflect patient concerns (for 'nice doctors') as opposed to professional concerns (for 'reduced prescribing rates').*

Like most patients I hold the NHS in high regard. I put enormous trust in my family practitioner. I share my personal and family history with him and I entrust my children's health to him. In return I expect primarily that no harm will come to my family because of his treatment. Trust is at the heart of the relationship and that is why the public is so shocked by incidents such as Bristol.

Primary care is a public service responding very largely to public demand. In an age of consumerism and government charter, practitioners in primary care have had to adjust to new demands for responsiveness, accessibility, quality and service. The debate now is not so much whether patients should be involved, but how. As with other aspects of clinical governance, for example risk reduction, there is much to learn from the techniques employed by commercial service industries.[1] They steadfastly avoid tokenism; learn constantly from customer feedback, especially complaints; and use a range of proactive methods for giving and receiving information, for example focus groups, customer panels and so on.

Arguably there has been a progressive adjustment in the balance (of power) between patient and professional in the context of consultation in primary care. For clinical governance to be effective this now needs to be expanded and extended to the other levels of the organisation. The lay members of primary care groups and trusts are well placed to help, but primary care groups will need to avoid falling into the trap of assuming that their lay members can be left to 'do' public involvement. As with most other aspects of clinical governance an actively multidisciplinary approach will be required.

People

Primary care is a people business, and the quality of care provided depends critically on adequate numbers of caring, competent and motivated staff, and the ability of those staff to work well in a team. There is a danger that, in an effort to ensure that practice is safe and effective, complex and time-consuming monitoring systems are developed rather than focusing on developing the people, their clinical practice and teamworking – teamworking where relationships are based on openness and trust within a clear framework of accountability.

There are important technical aspects of 'human resource management' (and training issues, e.g. nurse prescribing), which go beyond the scope of this book. Nevertheless, primary care organisations are going to need to get to grips with such matters as workforce planning, skill mix, occupational health, and the proper procedures for recruitment, selection, appraisal and discipline of staff. For example, in one of the most notorious untoward incidents in the health service in recent years (the Amanda Jenkinson case), much hinged on the accuracy of references in support of job applications and who had the authority and training to write them.[11]

The continuing professional development of staff (Chapter 12) and the development of leadership (Chapter 13) are covered elsewhere, but there are three important and related areas which merit discussion here – scope of professional practice, clinical supervision and professional self-regulation.

Scope of professional practice

Over the last two decades GPs have taken on a range of new roles, both in clinical care, e.g. minor surgery, care of patients with diabetes, and in the management of the health service, e.g. GP fundholding, commissioning. They have done so without recourse to a higher authority, and sometimes express frustration at their nursing colleagues' apparent inability to do the same at their behest!

In 1992 the regulatory body for nurses, the United Kingdom Central Council for Nursing, Midwifery and Health Visiting (UKCC), published *The Scope of Professional Practice*.[12] This replaced the 'extended role of the nurse' provision by which medical staff delegated tasks to nurses and had to certify the nurses' competence. The aim was to allow nurses to undertake new and expanding roles while continuing to safeguard public safety. The document asserted that 'each nurse is accountable for their own practice and that it is their professional judgement which can provide innovative solutions to meeting the needs of patients and clients in a health service that is constantly changing'.

Any nurse then can take on responsibilities outside their traditional role providing they adhere to the following principles. Nurses taking on new roles must:

- be satisfied that patient needs are uppermost
- aim to keep up-to-date and develop personal skills and competence
- recognise the limits to their personal knowledge and skill and remedy any deficiencies
- ensure that existing nursing care is not compromised by taking on new developments and responsibilities
- acknowledge personal accountability
- avoid inappropriate delegation.

This approach has allowed much greater flexibility and creativity in the development of nursing practice in response to patient needs, without nurses having to collect endless certificates. It does, however, place the onus on the practitioner to define the limits of their competence within the overall *Code of Professional Conduct*.

In its review of the impact of this change of policy, the UKCC identified many examples of innovative practice supported by the new flexibility on offer. These examples included midwifery-led maternity units, nurse triage, and nurse-led services in oncology, asthma care and a wide range of other areas. The expansion of *NHS Direct* and other nurse-led services is becoming increasingly important for primary care. The clinical governance of these services will rely heavily on the proper development of any extension of nurses' roles. It is likely that GPs will need to consider the same issues as revalidation becomes established.

Clinical supervision

Clinical supervision is normal professional practice for a number of the 'caring' professions, e.g. counsellors, psychotherapists. It has been defined as 'a formal process of professional support and learning which enables individual practitioners to develop knowledge and competence, assume responsibility for their own practice, and enhance consumer protection and safety in complex clinical situations'.[13] In essence it involves protected time for the practitioner(s), either individually or in a group, with a supervisor. The time is used in a structured way to reflect on practice; to review critical incidents; and to identify means of personal and practice development. Many practitioners, of course, have established informal means of supervision. The development of formal clinical supervision builds on the best of these by adding structure and commitment to the process.

Despite being formally endorsed by the UKCC in 1996,[14] the development of clinical supervision in nursing remains patchy, with disciplines such as midwifery and psychiatric nursing leading the way. It is virtually absent among GPs. The concept of supervision, however, has gained in popularity over recent years with the recognition that well-structured supervision can both improve the quality of service and, importantly, relieve stress on individual practitioners. Practitioners in primary care commonly encounter emotionally difficult situations, and yet have few formal methods for debriefing.

There is obviously a link between clinical supervision and clinical governance, and it has been suggested that active participation in clinical supervision is a clear demonstration of an individual exercising their responsibility under clinical governance.[15] The same authors, however, make the point that supervision needs to take place in the context of an overall framework, and not as an isolated activity.

In many ways supervision is the clinical equivalent of appraisal, and such mechanisms are sorely needed in primary care. For example, GPs working in partnership may (rarely) be able to engage in peer appraisal. Single-handed doctors, however, benefit from neither formal nor informal review by either peer or supervisor. This will be a major challenge for primary care groups and trusts.

Professional self-regulation

Professional self-regulation is one major element contributing to the quality assurance of NHS healthcare.[16] Whereas clinical governance might be said to apply to services, which are provided collectively, professional self-regulation is concerned with the fitness of individuals to practise. The government, and others, have argued that effective clinical governance needs enhanced professional regulation, and important changes are under way.

The UKCC is the nurses' equivalent of the GMC, and is responsible for the registration of nurses and for maintaining the standards of the profession. One of the key vehicles for achieving this is the *Code of Professional Conduct*,[17] which is reviewed and updated regularly. The code requires each registered nurse, midwife and health visitor to act at all times in such a manner as to:

- safeguard and promote the interests of individual patients and clients
- serve the interests of society
- justify public confidence
- uphold and enhance the good standing and reputation of the professions.

The UKCC's Professional Registration and Practice (PREP) requirements were introduced in 1995,[18] and formalised for the first time a requirement for continuing professional development. Under this each nurse must undertake a minimum of five days of study every three years, and maintain a personal professional profile detailing professional development. This process is of relevance to doctors as the GMC begins to introduce revalidation.

There has been much misinformation within the profession about PREP, with many courses offering 'PREP points' for nurses (not unlike PGEA accreditation for courses attended by GPs). Significantly, PREP was never intended to be about attending courses or collecting points. Rather it was meant to demonstrate continued development through involvement in a wide range of activities, which might include shadowing, undertaking clinical audit, a personal research project, or undertaking a literature review, as well as formal training.

The 'professional profile' is used to record all the information about career progress and professional development. It should be based on a regular process of reflection on learning from everyday experiences as well as planned learning activity. It is not a curriculum vitae, a daily diary or a life history, but a flexible and comprehensive account of professional development. There is no standard format for building profiles, but essentially there are three steps – reviewing experience to date, self-appraisal and goal setting with action plans. The process has potential value not only for nurses, but for other professional groups as well. Of more general importance it also services a key regulatory function for the profession of nursing. At present nurses must indicate that they have met the requirements as part of triennial re-registration. From April 2001 a sample of profiles will be audited to ensure standards are being met.

The late 1990s witnessed a watershed in the regulation of the medical profession, in many ways as historic as the passage of the first Medical Act in 1848. That act established the medical register and was intended to protect the public from charlatans. Only qualified medical practitioners were accepted on to the register. For the next 150 years doctors, once on the register, were not obliged to provide further evidence of their continuing fitness to practise. At its meetings in November 1998 and February 1999, however, the GMC endorsed key recommendations for the implementation of revalidation for all registered doctors. The Council agreed that specialists and GPs 'must be able to demonstrate – on a regular basis – that they are keeping themselves up to date and remain fit to practise in their chosen field'. This is the definition of revalidation.[19]

The GMC revalidation steering group did not attempt to design a detailed process for revalidation. They did, however, construct a simple framework, identifying six key stages in the process, to satisfy themselves that revalidation could be made to work (*see* Box 2.3). Of these stages only the requirement to provide the GMC with evidence of continuing fitness to practise was completely new. The similarity with PREP is obvious. The steering group further illustrated how the profiles of a doctor's practice could be based on data showing:

- a record of continuing educational activity
- a portfolio of wider professional development
- a record of participation in, and the results of, clinical and organisational audit
- the results of the regular appraisals which should reflect the above, showing any changes in the doctor's performance and be set in the context of national professional standards.

Box 2.3:   The six stages of GMC revalidation for doctors[19]

i   Local profiling of performance.
ii   Periodic external peer review of the profiling process.
iii   Providing evidence that would lead to revalidation of the doctor's entry in the register.

These three stages would apply to all doctors. Where there were concerns about a doctor's performance, one or more of the following would then be activated:

iv   Local remediation.
v   Referral to the GMC Performance Procedures.
vi   Action by the GMC on the doctor's registration.

The need for a system of regular appraisal, clinical supervision, has never been more pressing for GPs. Indeed it is needed for everyone working in primary care.

Processes

Clinical governance depends on the deployment of a coherent range of processes, many of which are described in the following chapters. There are, however, two important areas not covered elsewhere which deserve mention – accreditation and the protection of patient information.

Accreditation

There is a growing interest in accreditation, as a form of composite measure of quality assurance for primary care organisations. Accreditation has been defined as 'a system of external peer review for determining compliance with a set of standards'.[20] It involves a review of an organisation's performance by external agents. Performance is measured against a set of agreed criteria and explicit standards, and a report of the results is provided to the organisation. Accreditation can be used for a variety of purposes, but the examples in primary care are mainly focused on quality improvement (*see* Box 2.4).[21,22]

Box 2.4:   Accreditation programmes in primary care[21,22]

Health Quality Service Award	King's Fund (formerly known as Organisational Audit)
Training practices	Joint Committee on Postgraduate Training in General Practice (JCPTGP)
Membership by assessment of performance (MAP)	Royal College of General Practitioners
Team-based practice accreditation programme	Royal College of General Practitioners
Fellowship by assessment (FBA)	Royal College of General Practitioners
Quality practice award (QPA)	Royal College of General Practitioners
ISO 9000 (formerly BS 5750)	British Standards Institute
Investors in People	Training and Enterprise Councils
Charter Mark	Public Services
Benchmarking	NHS Estates

More information on these is available in *Quality Assessment in General Practice: supporting clinical governance in primary care groups* by Martin Roland and colleagues from the National Primary Care Research and Development Centre at Manchester University. www.npcrdc.man.ac.uk

---

In their evaluation of accreditation in primary care, Walsh and Walshe[21] suggest a number of questions that primary care organisations should ask before embarking on any particular scheme.

1   Purpose – is the primary purpose quality improvement, and how clear are the objectives?
2   Participation – is participation voluntary, and how many organisations have participated in the past?
3   Standards – at what level are the standards set, and how were they developed? What do they cover, and how are they measured?
4   Assessment methods – which data are needed? Who are the external assessors, and how were they selected and trained?
5   Presentation of results – how is the feedback to be provided, and is it confidential to the organisation?

6   Impact and follow-up – what is known of the effects on other organisations that have been accredited, and how will the process be followed up?
7   Costs – what are the fees charged, and what are the opportunity costs in terms of time and preparation?

A programme of accreditation for the primary care teams in a primary care group could prove a useful mechanism for the development of clinical governance. It would certainly provide opportunities for consistent external review across teams.

Protection of patient information

It is recognised that the improper disclosure of information about identifiable patients would undermine public confidence in the NHS. The protection of patient confidentiality is therefore a part of clinical governance, and NHS organisations 'will be held accountable, through clinical governance for continually improving confidentiality and security procedures' in line with the recommendations of the Caldicott Committee.[23]

All NHS organisations are required to appoint Caldicott Guardians, although in primary care there should be a single guardian for each primary care group, and within each practice a nominated lead person for confidentiality and security issues. The guardian should be, in order of priority:

•   an existing member of the management board of the organisation
•   a senior health professional
•   an individual with responsibility for promoting clinical governance within the organisation.

The guardians are intended to be responsible for agreeing and reviewing protocols governing both the protection and use of patient-identifiable information within their organisation, and disclosure of information across organisational boundaries. This appears a mighty task for any primary care group, and is described here for the sake of completeness.

Conclusion

There are two questions commonly asked by primary care staff. What is clinical governance? And what is my role in it? The first two chapters should have gone some way to answering the first of these questions. The answer to the second depends to some extent on the role of the individual.

The clinical governance lead for a primary care team or group will oversee and direct the many processes that contribute to clinical governance in their organisation. They cannot do it all themselves, and they cannot do it all at once. This will be a programme of development over some years.

For the practitioner, be they doctor, nurse or other professional, there is the responsibility for demonstrating their individual fitness to practise (revalidation or re-registration), as well as contributing to the collective quality assurance of the service provided to patients (clinical governance).

Practical points

- There is increasing pressure for greater accountability for the quality of primary care.
- Unacceptable variations in quality are evident.
- There has been fragmentation of the many initiatives aimed at quality improvement.
- Useful existing activities and resources can be built on.
- Early involvement of patients and carers should be considered.
- Primary care staff need support through mechanisms like appraisal and clinical supervision.
- All practitioners will have to demonstrate their fitness to practise on a periodic and regular basis.
- Collective clinical governance depends on the deployment of a coherent range of processes.
- Accreditation is a composite quality measure for an organisation, and has been used in primary care.

References

1   van Zwanenberg T (1998) GP tomorrow. In: J Harrison and T van Zwanenberg (eds) *GP Tomorrow*. Radcliffe Medical Press, Oxford.

2   Smith R (1998) All changed, changed utterly. *BMJ*. **316**: 1917–18.

3   Hunter D (1998) A case of under-management. *Health Services Journal*. 25 June: 18–19.

4   van Zwanenberg T (1998) Strategic shifts. In: J Harrison and T van Zwanenberg (eds) *GP Tomorrow*. Radcliffe Medical Press, Oxford.

5   Thomson R (1998) Quality to the fore in health policy – at last. *BMJ*. **317**: 95–6.

6   Houghton G (1997) From audit to effectiveness: an historical evaluation of the changing role of Medical Audit Advisory Groups. *Journal of Evaluation in Clinical Practice*. **3**,4: 245–53.

7   Department of Health (1997) *The New NHS: modern, dependable*. Cm 3807. The Stationery Office, London.

8   Department of Health (1999) *Clinical Governance: quality in the new NHS*. Health Service Circular: HSC(99)065. Department of Health, London.

9   Baker R, Lakhani M, Fraser R and Cheater F (1999) A model for clinical governance in primary care groups. *BMJ*. **318**: 779–83.

10   van Zwanenberg T (1998) *Clinical governance in primary care. Getting started – discussion paper*. Report for Health Authorities in the Tyne and Wear Health Action Zone.

11   North Nottingham Health Authority (1997) *Report of the independent inquiry into the major employment and ethical issues arising from the events leading to the trial of Amanda Jenkinson* (The Bullock Report), North Nottingham Health Authority, Bassetlaw.

12   UKCC (1992) *The Scope of Professional Practice*. UKCC, London.

13   Department of Health (1993) *A Vision for the Future*. Department of Health, London.

14   UKCC (1996) *Position Statement on Clinical Supervision for Nursing and Health Visiting*. UKCC, London.

15   Butterworth A and Woods D (1999) *Clinical Governance and Clinical Supervision: working together to ensure safe and effective practice*. University of Manchester, Manchester.

16   Secretary of State for Health (1998) *A First Class Service: quality in the NHS*. Stationery Office, London.

17   UKCC (1992) *Code of Professional Practice*. UKCC, London.

18   UKCC (1997) *PREP and You*. UKCC, London.

19   General Medical Council's Revalidation Steering Group (1999) *Report of the Revalidation Steering Group*. GMC, London.

20   Scrivens E (1995) *Accreditation: protecting the professional or the consumer?* Open University Press, Buckingham.

21   Walsh N and Walshe K (1998) *Accreditation in Primary Care*. Health Services Management Centre, University of Birmingham.

22   Roland R, Holden J and Campbell S (1999) *Quality Assessment for General Practice: supporting clinical governance in primary care groups*. National Primary Care Research and Development Centre, University of Manchester.

23   Department of Health (1999) *Caldicott Guardians*. Health Service Circular: HSC(99)012. Department of Health, London.

Clinical governance in practice

CHAPTER THREE

What are patients looking for?

Marianne Rigge

This chapter describes how most patients are experts in their own right, and good judges of the quality of healthcare. Primary care groups need to develop skills to engage, understand and interpret the views of patients.

One of the most welcome statements in the government's quality consultation paper, *A First Class Service*, must surely have been 'We need to move away from merely counting numbers ... clinical governance will help to ensure that quality resumes its rightful place at the heart of the NHS'.[1]

Unfortunately the document failed to define quality. We *were* told, however, in the White Paper *The New NHS*, who the experts will be. 'Primary care professionals are identified as best placed to understand their patients' needs as a whole and to identify ways of making services more responsive'.[2] And the same document identified community health services as 'being able to take account of the special needs of black and ethnic minority patients and to draw attention to the wider health needs of the community'.

When putting together our response to the White Paper, the College of Health was collectively dismayed by an editorial in the magazine *GP*, clearly supporting the idea that doctor knows best, while putting us silly patients firmly in our place.

'The public's grasp of complex health issues can be tenuous, and explaining the issues will absorb the time and resources of primary care groups. Those GPs involved in the process ... are faced with the more pressing issues of commissioning care.'[3]

Other commentators have gone so far as to say that the patients' contribution in *The New NHS* is relegated to a poor second, even third, place and that there is a real danger of signalling a return to the paternalistic attitudes that have been so heavily criticised in the past.[4]

That remains to be seen. But it is clear that there is much to be done if patients' views and needs are genuinely to be taken on board, rather than be assumed by those who are deemed to know best. The tokenistic appointment of sole lay representatives to primary care groups does not exactly suggest that we are going in the right direction.

If we are to achieve a genuine engagement with users of health services as patients and carers, and as user representatives and advocates from the wealth of self-help and voluntary groups, we need first to acknowledge that many health professionals are unused to seeking out patients' views. Nor can we assume that even those who are willing to try, will have the skills to engage, understand and correctly interpret those views.

How do you find out what makes a quality service from the patient's point of view? The answer is simple, though not simplistic. You ask the patient. Over the last decade or so, the College of Health has carried out well over 50 studies designed to find out about patients' views and experiences of virtually every aspect of the health service. We use a range of qualitative research techniques which we call 'consumer audit', including, for example, focus groups. We have published a number of guides on how to go about this which have been commended by the NHS Executive.[5–7] We offer training courses in qualitative research methods and in how to be effective in the new role of lay member of a primary care group (*see* section on sources of information and help).

What all our studies have shown is that many patients are experts in their own right. They make good judges of the quality of every dimension of healthcare, including access and process, but most importantly outcome, as the following quotes from real patients demonstrate. They took part in a ground-breaking study carried out by the College of Health for the Royal College of Physicians to help develop a methodology for producing patient-centred guidelines for rehabilitation after stroke.[8] We conducted a similar study with people who have rheumatoid arthritis (RA).[9] Both suggest that GPs and the rest of the primary care team should be more alert to patients' needs for much better information, advice, support and guidance towards other sources of help to improve the quality of their lives. This could be a vastly important role for the new primary care groups and the primary care trusts which will follow. But only if they find ways of tapping into the views and needs of their patients, as well as their unpaid carers – without whom the NHS would certainly collapse.

> *The practice is very, very busy. Even with personal problems, you still feel you are being rushed in and rushed out as quickly as possible. It's very different from the practice I grew up with, where the family doctor knew the whole family and knew all of their problems. He was more of a friend.*

Good communication, or the lack of it, are constantly recurring themes, as is the need for much more information.

> *You'd phone the doctor any time you needed, and he came immediately. My husband was pretty ill. He still is. But if there's a problem, I know the doctor will come. He's very good. It's good to be able to talk to him with all the problems ... he gives the time to listen ... he gives me good support. (Stroke patient carer)*

What's wrong is that doctors don't know enough about strokes or what it's like to be a stroke victim. You go to any surgery and they've got groups for diabetics, they've got groups for asthma, groups for arthritis. But there's not groups for stroke victims because the doctors don't know themselves. It took me years to find out about the Stroke Association and when I think of all the help they could have given me when I really needed it, at my lowest ebb...

These attacks, they used to last for hours. They were very frightening and at the end I couldn't move. The doctor didn't seem to appreciate that I really was ill. All he could do was prescribe ever more steroids ... But he retired and our new doctor referred me straight away and the rheumatologist was very stunned at the amount of steroids I'd had, and they'd done a lot of damage. (RA patient)

One of the main lessons we have learnt through such studies is that it is vital to let the patient or carer set the agenda, whether in a focus group or a one-to-one interview. This is especially the case with people from marginalised groups and those with special and complex needs, such as people with learning difficulties and mental health service users. They too are often faced with fragmented health and social services which do not necessarily talk to one another, despite all the rhetoric about seamless care.

Primary care groups and trusts could really come into their own if they gave a proper place to meaningful consultation with their very different patient and client groups. Those best placed to orchestrate this may well not be GPs but, for instance, community psychiatric nurses and colleagues from other community and mental health services.

Primary care groups need also to think long and hard about the way some of their patients are typecast as 'heartsink' or 'inappropriate attenders' at accident and emergency departments, when the reality may be that it is their doctors who are heartsink – elderly, single-handed, working from sub-standard, lock-up premises in dangerous parts of the inner city, where no one in their right mind would turn up in the middle of the night hoping for a diagnosis of meningitis in their small child or even the simplest treatment.

If there is a real window of opportunity to be grasped by the proposals set out in the *The New NHS* and *A First Class Service*, it must lie somewhere in the institution of primary care groups and trusts, linked with strong primary care audit (ultimately clinical governance) groups.

The reason for this is that GPs and other members of the primary care team are not just the gatekeepers to the rest of the system, they are also the pickers up of pieces. They hold the key to identifying the things that can go wrong when their patients fall between the net of the different strands of care. The College of Health has a dossier of examples of the suffering that can be caused by the very long periods that can elapse between referral to hospital and actually being seen by a consultant. These can be well over a year – and that's before they join the 18-month waiting list to be admitted under the Patient's Charter.[10]

During this time, they will be regarded as statistics to be counted, as trauma and orthopaedics or ophthalmology 'cases', not as real people who may develop ulcers because they have to take so many painkillers for their arthritic hip or knee, or who fall and fracture their femur because they can no longer see properly.

It is the primary care team that will be the first port of call for patients in such need and it is they who need to act as advocates on their behalf. It is also the primary care team that is in a position to follow the patient pathway, or journey through the health service and then to link outcomes to the range of interventions and procedures they undergo, as well as the length of time they have to wait for them.

There is a challenge here for audit groups and it is that they should start to pool resources and think big. If every primary care group were to agree to work with one another and genuinely share the information they glean, including information about things that do not work as they should, we could be well on the way to a revolution in the way the results of audit are put into practice.

But one more step is needed. Primary care audit groups need to work much more closely with patients, as well as their colleagues in the acute sector, and to share the results of their work. This new partnership needs to be built into all the systems now being set up for clinical governance. The unofficial new jargon for this type of initiative seems to be 'joined-up thinking'! In reality what it boils down to is intelligence and common sense and patient groups are not lacking in either of these.

As things are at present, there seems to be some sort of atavistic fear about sharing or publicising the results of audit. Of course, there are genuine and understandable reasons for clinicians to fear being identified when they are one among few, for example in a single primary healthcare team or acute service directorate, especially when litigation seems to be rising. And there is a corresponding and quite proper concern for patient confidentiality.

But that is the point. If clinical audit is shared and conducted on a much wider basis, there will be far less to fear in this respect. A more general point is that it is really not tenable to ask people to take part in research (and I include audit), if you are not prepared to share with them even the generalisable results.

This is particularly the case at a time of heightened public awareness of unacceptable mortality and morbidity, following such tragic events as unfolded at the Bristol Royal Infirmary or the Kent and Canterbury Hospitals Trust. Nor when it's becoming clear that cancer patients are still not necessarily being referred to an appropriate cancer specialist, despite the Calman–Hine recommendations and an awareness that the UK performs poorly in the international league tables of cancer mortality.[10]

At the College of Health, we have a long-standing concern about the lack of information to patients on consultants' qualifications, training and special interests. What is even more worrying, however, is a growing trend for hospitals not to supply such information to GPs. Our National Waiting List Helpline's most recent survey of every acute trust specifically asked for copies of information about consultants' special interests that they send to GPs. We were shocked to find that only half are supplying this to GPs, never mind patients, despite what it says in the Code of Practice on Openness in the NHS, which this government must surely sign up to.[11]

If clinical governance is about anything, it must be about openness and accountability, and primary care groups must insist on both if they are to play a major part in ironing out inefficiencies and inequalities in the system.

So what should primary care groups be doing?

Listen to National Institute for Clinical Excellence (NICE) but be proactive – NICE can't do everything

- Put nationally agreed guidelines into practice by developing robust protocols for clinical audit at the local level and involve patients and carers in the process.
- Make sure that patients and carers have access to patient versions of new guidelines as they are developed and encourage them to be interactive about the ways these are put into practice and reported on.
- Enter into a continuing dialogue with trust clinical directorates to ensure that referral protocols are in place which conform with patient-centred guidelines.
- Agree with colleagues about what diagnostic and other tests should be ordered, by whom and at what stage, as well as how, when and by whom the results should be communicated to patients.
- Agree protocols for pain relief and other symptom management, especially for those patients unable to take analgesics for iatrogenic and other reasons.
- Be aware of the need to guide patients towards sources of information, help and advice for coping with their illness and its effects, especially if they have to wait for extended periods before treatment can be carried out. This might include physiotherapy and occupational therapy, aids and adaptations available through social services, welfare and other benefits, or self-help groups and voluntary organisations. You are not expected to know about all of these through some process of osmosis. There are others out there who do (*see* section on sources of information and help).
- Remember that many patients do not present with 'evidence-based illnesses'. You know, better than most specialists, that many illnesses are multifactorial in causation and presentation, and that some may never be satisfactorily diagnosed. That is not to say that patients do not need and deserve the best standard of treatment and management of the uncertainty this gives rise to, which will probably be as distressing for you as it is for your patients. Certainly one of the downsides of the rapid rise in sub-specialisation is that there is now a dearth of the old-fashioned breed of physician whose wisdom may not have been evidence-based according to the new gold standards but remains much needed in 'difficult' cases.
- Insist on discharge protocols to ensure that patients receive the full range of information, advice and support when they are sent home, and that you are fully informed about what has been done to them, by whom and what follow-up is planned. You also need to know what your patients have been told and what their expectations are.
- Follow through your patients and devise systems for reporting back on what happens to them after discharge. Otherwise your hospital colleagues won't know what the final outcomes really were. Seeing a junior doctor in outpatients six weeks post-discharge does not suffice. They are likely to be ticked off as a 'successful outcome' because they have been discharged alive and have managed to get to their post-operative appointment in one piece!
- Bear in mind that a rigid insistence that guidelines must be based only on the evidence of scientific trials is unhelpful to patients. Medicine is an art as well as a

science and sometimes results will depend as much on patient compliance as on the treatment administered. This, in turn, may depend on the quality of communication with patients and the information they are given. Your hospital colleagues may fall short on this. It is not necessarily their fault since they probably won't have been taught much about this in medical school, and almost certainly not thereafter.

- Don't believe everything they say about randomised controlled trials being the gold standard. Vast numbers of procedures and treatments being carried out on your patients have never been subjected to these; for some it would not be possible. In any case, there is a recognised bias towards reporting only the results of those trials that have been successful and most of these will have ruled out people who might spoil the science because they are children, women of childbearing age, elderly, come from ethnic minorities or have other things the matter with them.
- Remember that an over-reliance on evidence-based guidelines may mean that patients suffering from conditions, or undergoing treatments, for which there is a lack of scientifically robust data, are denied information about what is current good or acceptable practice in the 'light' of known uncertainty.

Where do we go from here?

NICE may be part of the answer but it will not be a panacea. At the present rate of guideline development, we are many years away from being able to tell patients suffering from even some of the most common conditions, what sort of standard of treatment they should be able to expect. Where there is confusion and uncertainty, they deserve to be told that. What is needed is a more pragmatic and patient-centred approach. The people best placed to take that approach are the ones whom patients approach in the first place, the ones in whom they put their trust in what remains an intrinsically personal and most-favoured relationship. They don't deserve to be let down by squabbles about who should have most power in the new systems being imposed on this 'New' NHS of ours. Because it is all of ours and the ethos of compassion and care needs to prevail if we are to make the best of it. That's what patients will be looking for from clinical governance in primary healthcare.

Sources of information and help

Training

The College of Health offers a range of training workshops including:

- training for lay members of primary care groups: how to be effective in your new role
- training and support for lay representatives

- training in qualitative research methods including focus groups, qualitative inter-viewing techniques and qualitative analysis
- user-focused questionnaire design
- effective user involvement in health services.

Courses can also be run at your site as well as in London and other major cities. For further information contact:

Jessica Bush or Francesca Avbara at
The College of Health
St Margaret's House
21 Old Ford Road
London E2 9PL
020 8983 1225
020 8983 1553
e-mail jessica@tcoh.demon.co.uk

Self-help group database

Health data 2000

This database, programmed in Microsoft Access, contains details of over 2000 national health-related self-help groups.

Local health and self-help groups shell

The Health data 2000 Self-help Groups database can be provided with a shell to populate with your own local health information including local groups, health authority details, primary care details, NHS trusts, opticians, dentists, community pharmacies, clinics, etc.

Health information

Healthline tapes

The College of Health has produced over 500 audio tapes on health-related topics. Pro-fessionally recorded, they are designed to be listened to over the phone and thus available 24 hours a day. The information is regularly updated and validated by medical experts.

Healthline factsheets

Factsheets on over 500 health-related topics can be printed out from your computer to provide another valuable information resource for your patients. Using a question and answer format, the factsheets provide important basic information often including further sources of health and support.

Health Information Service

The Health Information Service is a national freephone service providing information on 0800 665544. The service can answer questions on local NHS services, self-help groups, diseases, conditions and treatments, how to complain as well as hospital waiting times and Charter standards.

Practical points

- Patients and carers are good judges of the quality of healthcare.
- There are well-described techniques for ascertaining the views of patients.
- Primary care groups should pool resources and share information, so that the results of audit are put into practice.
- Involve patients and carers in the process of implementing national guidelines from NICE, and make sure that they have patient versions of the guidelines.
- Work with secondary care clinicians and patients to sort out referral and discharge protocols.
- Guide patients towards sources of information, help and advice. These sources do exist. Primary care practitioners do not have to know it all.
- Many patients do not have 'evidence-based illnesses', but they still deserve the best standard of treatment, care and compassion.

References

1   Department of Health (1998) *A First Class Service: quality in the new NHS*. Health Service Circular: HSC(98)113. Department of Health, London.

2   Department of Health (1997) *The New NHS: modern, dependable*. Cm 3807. The Stationery Office, London.

3   Editorial (1998) Care needed with patient input. *General Practitioner.* 16 January 1999.

4   Rhodes P and Nocon A (1998) *User Involvement and the NHS Reforms. Health Expectations*. Blackwell Science, Oxford.

5   College of Health (1994) *Consumer Audit Guidelines.* College of Health, London.

6   Kelson M (1995) *Consumer Involvement Initiatives in Clinical Audit and Outcomes. A Review of Developments and Issues in the Identification of Good Practice*. College of Health, London.

7   Kelson M (1999) *Patient-defined outcomes*. Paper prepared on behalf of the Clinical Outcomes Group patient group. College of Health, London.

8   Kelson M, Rigge M and Ford C (1998) *Report on a College of Health and Royal College of Physicians Project Stroke Rehabilitation Patient and Carer Views.* Royal College of Physicians, London.

9   Rigge M (1998) Developing patient-centred guidelines for rheumatoid arthritis. *Guidelines in Practice.* **1**: 25–8.

10 Rigge M (1998) *College of Health Response to the NHS Consultative Paper, The New NHS: guidance on out of area treatment.* College of Health, London.

CHAPTER FOUR

Evidence-based practice

Ian Watt

This chapter describes a structured approach to evidence-based practice. The approach includes five steps – asking questions, tracking down the evidence, appraising the evidence, applying evidence-based practice and evaluating performance.

What is evidence-based practice?

Evidence-based healthcare is one of the key components of clinical governance. Unfortunately, the term has slipped into everyday usage with little common understanding of what it involves. Many misconceptions and prejudices have arisen around evidence-based practice, which those involved in clinical governance will need to overcome.

Whilst the philosophical origins of evidence-based practice have been said to date back to mid-19th century Paris and earlier, it is only since the early 1990s that its importance has been emphasised in the NHS. In 1991 the NHS Research and Development Strategy was launched with an aim to 'secure a knowledge-based health service in which clinical, managerial and policy decisions are based on sound and pertinent information'. Since then a number of different initiatives have been used to promote what has essentially been the same concept – evidence-based practice. Given the plethora of terms in use, it is worth clarifying definitions.

Sackett and colleagues have defined evidence-based medicine as

the conscientious, explicit and judicious use of current best evidence in making decisions about the care of individual patients.[1]

They go on to state that this means 'integrating individual clinical expertise, with the best available external clinical evidence from systematic research. This should be done in consultation with the patient in order to decide upon the option which suits that patient best'.

One of the criticisms levelled at evidence-based medicine is that it leads to so-called cookbook medicine. As defined above, however, there is a clear recognition of the importance of clinical expertise and individual patient factors in deciding whether and how external evidence should be applied to an individual. Slavish, cookbook approaches to individual patient care should be discouraged. Following on from Sackett *et al.*'s definition, the term 'evidence-based' has been applied to a number of areas in health and healthcare, for example, nursing, health promotion and policy making. For simplicity, the generic term evidence-based practice is used here.

Another term that is sometimes used interchangeably with evidence-based practice is clinical effectiveness. Formal definitions are given in Box 4.1, but more simply, an effective healthcare intervention can be defined as one that does more good than harm, and a cost-effective intervention as one doing more good than harm at least cost.

Box 4.1:   Some definitions

Evidence-based practice
The conscientious, explicit and judicious use of current best evidence in making decisions about the care of individual patients.

Effectiveness
The extent to which a specific intervention, procedure, regimen or service, when deployed in the field, does what it is intended to do for a defined population.

Efficacy
The extent to which a specific intervention, procedure, regimen or service produces a beneficial result under ideal conditions. Ideally, the determination of efficacy is based upon the results of a randomised controlled trial.

An approach to evidence-based practice

As evidence-based practice has developed, a more formal approach to its application has gained acceptance. This proposes five steps whereby answers to clinical questions are sought, appraised and applied in clinical practice (*see* Box 4.2).[2]

For the individual practitioner, evidence-based practice provides one approach to self-directed learning, where answers can be found for the diagnostic, prognostic and therapeutic problems presented by patients. Evidence-based practice also offers a framework for those practitioners with a responsibility for the quality of healthcare at a population level. For example, those involved in developing a clinical protocol, or guideline, for a primary care group, should seek to ensure that it is based on good evidence.

Box 4.2:   Steps in evidence-based practice

What does evidence-based practice involve?

1   Converting information needs into answerable questions.
2   Tracking down the best evidence with which to answer them.
3   Critically appraising that evidence for its validity (closeness to the truth) and usefulness
     (clinical applicability).
4   Applying the results of this appraisal to clinical practice.
5   Evaluating performance.

Whilst the steps outlined in Box 4.2 can appear overly rigid and time-consuming, they do provide a structured framework for the application of evidence in clinical practice. Not all have to be undertaken by the same person. Each of the stages is now considered in more detail.

Stage 1: asking questions

Clinical questions arise from individual clinical encounters and from the process of developing clinical policies and guidance. Practitioners can overestimate the extent and accuracy of their clinical knowledge, and are not always aware of the latest research findings. Inevitably, knowledge, and probably clinical performance, deteriorate with time. To prevent this, practitioners need to be prepared to reflect on their practice and question its appropriateness. Without this reflection, practice fails to benefit from research, and risks becoming out of date, leading to sub-optimal care for patients.

The process of clinical governance will need to ensure that practitioners can question their practice and that effective life-long learning is encouraged and supported. Evidence-based practice starts with identifying information needs and converting these into answerable questions. Often this is not as easy as it sounds. If questions are poorly constructed and/or too vague, it may not be possible to find the best evidence with which to answer them. To help focus such questions they should be based on four components:

(i)   the patient or problem
(ii)   the intervention
(iii) the comparison intervention (if relevant)
(iv)   the outcomes of interest.

For example:

(i)   in obese patients with Type 2 diabetes ...
(ii)   does metformin ...

(iii) compared with sulphonylureas ...
(iv) lead to improved diabetic control, lower all cause mortality and improve quality of life.

Stage 2: tracking down the evidence

Evidence, in a legal sense, may come from a number of sources. In the context of evidence-based practice, however, it should ideally come from high-quality scientific research. The most appropriate type of research study from which to glean the evidence will vary according to the nature of the question posed. For example, a question concerning the effectiveness of an intervention is normally best answered by a randomised controlled trial. This is because randomised controlled trials, if performed well, are the research design least susceptible to bias.

Even when undertaken correctly, some study designs are more susceptible than others to bias. For this reason hierarchies of evidence have been developed to help make judgements about the strength of the evidence available. One such hierarchy is shown in Box 4.3, with the most reliable designs (with respect to answering questions of effectiveness) at the top. The least reliable evidence on clinical effectiveness comes from expert opinion.

Box 4.3:   Hierarchy of evidence

1   Evidence from systematic reviews of multiple, well-designed, randomised controlled trials.
2   Evidence from at least one properly designed, randomised controlled trial of appropriate size.
3   Evidence from well-designed, non-randomised trials, non-controlled intervention studies, cohort studies, time series or case–control studies.
4   Evidence from well-designed, non-experimental studies from more than one centre or research group.
5   Opinions of respected authorities based on clinical experience, descriptive studies and reports of expert committees.

This is not to imply that randomised controlled trials can be used to answer all healthcare questions. For example, they may not always be feasible because of cost or ethical considerations.

Another research design which is useful in evidence-based practice is the systematic review (*see* Box 4.4).[3] These differ from ordinary reviews in following an explicit method and seeking to be as objective as possible. Given the increasing amount of new research

---

Box 4.4:   Systematic reviews

Review – the general term for all attempts to synthesise the results and conclusions of two or more publications on a given topic.

Systematic review – a comprehensive review which strives to identify and track down all the literature on a topic (also called systematic literature review).

Meta-analysis – a technique which incorporates a specific statistical strategy for assembling the results of several studies into a single estimated overall result.

---

evidence (over 2 000 000 articles published annually in over 20 000 biomedical journals), systematic reviews can provide reliable summaries of research evidence, and are particularly useful for busy practitioners in primary care.

Sources of evidence

It is a salutary fact that only a small proportion of the vast quantity of research published each year is of high quality. In addition, the reliable evidence may be scattered across many different journals. Electronic databases such as Medline and Embase can help identify relevant studies, but searching them is not always easy. Because of inadequacies in the indexing of research papers, even the best searchers may fail to find relevant studies. In general, only about half of the randomised controlled trials in Medline can be found by even the best electronic searcher.[4] In addition, electronic databases are not exhaustive in their coverage, with Medline, for example, covering only about 6000 of the 20 000 journals published worldwide.

Potential solutions to these problems include:

- using good search strategies
- seeking systematic reviews to answer questions
- using specialised databases.

The help of an experienced librarian is often invaluable.

Search strategies

Identifying relevant research to meet a specific information need, can be optimised by using a tailored set of instructions for a particular database, in order to give the richest yield of relevant studies. Information on designing effective search strategies is given in Box 4.5.

Box 4.5:   Helpful information on search strategies

Electronic sources of advice include:

Predefined search strategies to locate systematic reviews on Medline and CINAHL are available at the web site of the NHS Centre for Reviews and Dissemination: http://www.york.ac.uk/inst/crd/search.htm

A range of strategies including search strategies to locate randomised controlled trials can be found at http://www.ihs.ox.ac.uk/library/filters.html

Search strategies are available via the PubMED free Medline site: http://www.ncbi.nlm.nih.gov/PubMed/clinical.html

Further reading

- Muir Gray JA (1997) *Evidence-based Healthcare*. Churchill Livingstone, Edinburgh.
- Glanville J (1999) Carrying out the literature search. In: S Curran and CJ Williams (eds) *Clinical Research in Psychiatry*. Butterworth-Heinemann, Oxford.

Systematic reviews

Because good systematic reviews will have tracked down and appraised most of the relevant high-quality research on a specific area of concern, they undoubtedly represent the best starting point for answering clinical questions. In the past, good systematic reviews were few and far between. They are now becoming an increasingly popular research tool applied to a wide range of clinical areas. Their quality is also improving.

Perhaps the most influential group in this respect is the Cochrane Collaboration – an international research initiative set up to produce, maintain and disseminate systematic reviews of the research evidence relevant to health and healthcare. Cochrane reviews can be found in the Cochrane Library (*see* Box 4.6), a regularly updated electronic library of related databases.

Also in the Cochrane Library (and available on-line in its own right) is another source of high-quality systematic reviews – the Database of Abstracts of Reviews of Effectiveness (DARE). This is produced by the NHS Centre for Reviews and Dissemination (CRD) at the University of York and consists of abstracts of quality-assessed systematic reviews, together with critical commentaries written by York researchers. CRD also produced a similar database of economic evaluations – the NHS Economic Evaluation Database (NHS EED) which can be used to help answer questions related to cost-effectiveness.

Specialist databases

Medline is probably the electronic database most familiar to health professionals and is a useful resource. However, because of the problems of limited coverage of published journals

---

Box 4.6:   Helpful sources of systematic reviews

The Cochrane Library – a regularly updated electronic library containing:

- The Cochrane Database of Systematic Reviews – full text of reviews produced and updated by the Cochrane Collaboration.
- The Database of Abstracts of Reviews of Effectiveness (DARE) produced by the NHS Centre for Reviews and Dissemination, University of York, contains structured summaries of quality assessed reviews produced by non-Cochrane researchers.
- The Cochrane Controlled Trials Register – a bibliography of over 100 000 controlled trials.
- The Cochrane Review Methodology Database – a bibliography of articles on undertaking systematic reviews.

The Cochrane Library is available on CD-ROM (to subscribe contact Update Software, PO Box 696, Oxford OX2 7YX) and via the internet (http://www.update-software.com/ccweb/cochrane/cdsr.htm)

The NHS Centre for Reviews and Dissemination, University of York

A facility commissioned by the NHS Research and Development Programme to undertake, commission and identify reviews on the effectiveness and cost-effectiveness of health interventions, and disseminate them to the NHS. It produces:

- DARE – see above. Also free on-line.
- NHS Economic Evaluation Database – structured summaries of economic evaluations. Available free on-line.
- Effective Health Care Bulletins – a bi-monthly bulletin in which the effectiveness of a variety of healthcare interventions is examined, based on a systematic review and synthesis of research on clinical effectiveness, cost-effectiveness and acceptability. It is distributed widely free of charge throughout the NHS, including all general practices and postgraduate libraries.
- Effectiveness Matters – bulletins with short summaries of systematic reviews with important messages for the NHS. A similar distribution to the Effective Health Care Bulletins.

Information on CRD or its products can be obtained via University of York, York YO1 5DD; e-mail revdis@york.ac.uk. CRD databases can be searched via their web pages: http://nhscrd.york.ac.uk/welcome.html

---

and inadequate indexing of research papers, it may not be the most effective way of meeting specialised information needs or finding specific types of research, such as systematic reviews. Hence, it is always worth asking a librarian about the existence of databases specialising in research in the specified area of interest. With respect to specific types of research study, for example randomised controlled trials and systematic reviews, the Cochrane Library should normally be the first database to consult.

Stage 3: appraising the evidence

Having tracked down the research information, the next step is to assess its validity, i.e. to make an assessment of how 'true' the study conclusions are. Two aspects of validity are normally assessed: internal validity, where an assessment is made of how likely it is that the study conclusions are biased due to inadequacies in study design or analysis; and external validity (reliability), where a judgement is made of how far the study conclusions can be generalised to circumstances other than those found in the original research.

It is not within the scope of this chapter to provide detailed advice on the assessment of the validity of research studies. It is important to stress, however, that research conclusions should not be adopted without some appraisal of the studies from which they have been drawn. Such appraisal is often helped by following a checklist of questions so that all the important issues of design, analysis and interpretation can be assessed. Sources of advice on critical appraisal, including useful checklists, are given in Box 4.7.

Box 4.7:   **Some examples of helpful information on critical appraisal**

- Crombie IK (1996) *The Pocket Guide to Critical Appraisal*. BMJ Publishing, London.
- Sackett DL, Haynes RB, Guyatt GTT, *et al.* (1991) *Clinical Epidemiology*. Little Brown, Boston, MA.
- Users' Guides to the Medical Literature prepared by the Evidence-Based Medicine Working Group are available on the World Wide Web at: http://hiru.mcmaster.ca/ebm/userguid/
- How to read a paper. A series of articles written by T. Greenhalgh providing a good overview of basic critical appraisal. Published in the *British Medical Journal* in eight weekly articles starting *BMJ* (1997) **315**: 180–3; also now in a book: Greenhalgh T (1998) *How to Read a Paper*. BMJ Publishing, London.
- Chambers R (1998) *Clinical Effectiveness Made Easy. First Thoughts on Clinical Governance*. Radcliffe Medical Press, Oxford.

Increasingly, there are now sources of research-based information becoming available where someone else has appraised the validity of the studies. These assessments, undertaken by those with expertise in critical appraisal, are useful for busy practitioners who may have neither the time nor the skills to undertaken detailed appraisals themselves.

Sources of appraised research information are given in Box 4.8. As already indicated, systematic reviews are useful in this respect, as the reviewer will have had to appraise all

---

Box 4.8:   Some examples of sources of appraised research evidence

- *Evidence Based Medicine* – a bimonthly journal which identifies and appraises high-quality, clinically relevant research. The articles are summarised in informative abstracts and commented on by clinical experts. For further information: http://www.bmjpg.com/data/ebm.htm
- *ACP Journal Club* – related to *Evidence Based Medicine* and published by the American College of Physicians. Abstracts restricted to internal medicine: http://www.acponline.org/journals/acpjc/jcmenu.htm
- *Evidence Based Nursing*: http://www.bmjpg.com/data/ebn.htm
- *Evidence Based Mental Health*: http://www.psychiatry.ox.ac.uk/cebmh/journal/index.html
- *Evidence Based Health Policy and Management*: http://www.ihs.ox.ac.uk/ebhpm/index.html
- *Bandolier* – a monthly newsletter published by the NHS. Aims to produce up-to-date information on the effectiveness of healthcare interventions: http://www.jr2.ox.ac.uk/Bandolier
- *Drug and Therapeutics Bulletin* – an independent review of the effectiveness of mainly pharmacological interventions produced by the Consumers' Association: http://www.which.net
- *Clinical Evidence* – a twice-yearly compendium of evidence on the benefits and harms of common clinical interventions: http://www.evidence.org

---

the relevant primary research. Unfortunately, systematic reviews can also be prone to bias like any other research method, and should not be interpreted uncritically.

Stage 4: applying evidence-based practice

For clinical governance to succeed, the principles at least behind the steps outlined above will need to be understood by all primary care staff. Given that this will not be achieved easily, it is reasonable to ask 'why bother?'. Three main reasons can be given.

(i)   Medical knowledge is changing at a rapid rate. The notion that the body of knowledge at completion of professional training remains unchanged throughout a clinical career is simply untenable.

(ii) The sheer volume of health-related research and the wide variation in its quality makes it increasingly easy to miss valid research, which could benefit patient care.

(iii) Patients are becoming much better informed about all aspects of their healthcare, through sources such as magazines, television and more recently, the internet.

Whilst the information they gather may not always be valid, patients do want to discuss the options for their healthcare and they expect their practitioners to be well-informed.

The rationale for evidence-based practice is thus well-founded, but its widespread application in primary care raises a number of issues.

Finding the time and other resources

Almost every clinical encounter generates the need for further information for the practitioner. In addition, clinical guidelines are becoming increasingly popular in the drive to improve the quality of healthcare. There is a danger that practitioners could become swamped in the process of tracking down, appraising and applying the answers to all their clinical questions. For most clinicians, time is the major barrier and they will need to prioritise their information needs. Busy clinicians may find the following criteria helpful:

* the importance of the question to the patient's care
* the feasibility of answering the question in the time available
* the interest of the clinician in the problem
* the questions most lkely to provide answers which help other patients.

Those charged with the development of evidence-based guidelines will also need to prioritise the topics addressed. If primary care is overloaded with guidelines, they will not be implemented effectively, being left to gather dust on some forgotten shelf.

In addition to time, evidence-based practice also requires access to relevant sources of research information. A good postgraduate library service is important, but is no substitute for decent resources at practice level. Practices need to have good information facilities of their own. In particular, they should have access to electronic media, such as the internet, and to databases, such as the Cochrane Library.

A lack of evidence

Primary care practitioners see an extremely wide range of clinical problems and presentations. A consequence of this is that the research with which to answer a particular clinical question may not have been undertaken. Even where the research exists, it may have been undertaken in circumstances that caution against its application in primary care. To safeguard internal validity, researchers often control the types of patients recruited to studies.

For example, a study of the efficacy of a new antihypertensive drug might include only men aged under 65 years with no co-morbidities. This makes it difficult to generalise the study conclusions to the wide variety of patients seen in primary care. There are further problems of generalisability. Much of the research is undertaken in secondary care, where the patients do not necessarily possess the same characteristics as those with the same condition in the wider community.

These issues, however, should not prevent evidence-based practice from being carried out in primary care. They highlight the need for a critical approach, and for more research to be undertaken in primary care. And there still remains a large volume of evidence that can usefully be applied in the primary care setting.[5]

The public

The public are becoming better informed about many aspects of healthcare. This can act as a spur to evidence-based practice, particularly when patients want an informed discussion about their care. The discussion of research evidence with lay people inevitably requires a certain skill to explain and interpret the findings. Practitioners need to gauge patients' level of understanding, the amount of information they require and the desired level of involvement in decision-making. Much of the publicly accessible health information is of good quality, but some is not. Practitioners may need to appraise information jointly with the patient. An informed public should not be viewed as a threat, although it does make it harder for practitioners to avoid taking an evidence-based approach.

Stage 5: evaluating performance

The final part of the evidence-based practice pathway involves assessing whether research recommendations have been implemented and what impact they have had on patients outcomes. For the individual practitioner, a formal evaluation of whether the answers to all clinical questions assessed by this approach are implemented would be a daunting task. Nevertheless, this step emphasises that practical recommendations rarely get implemented without a conscious strategy.

In addition, once implemented, the improved patient outcomes predicted by the original research may not be realised if there are differences between the study conditions and practice. Practitioners should, at least, undertake regular informal evaluations of their implementation of evidence-based practice.

A number of more formal methods of monitoring performance are discussed elsewhere in this book (*see* Chapters 6 and 7). Clinical audit is probably the best known, and audit criteria and standards should be based on best evidence. Formal mechanisms to evaluate performance need to be restricted to priority topics, particularly those where large groups of patients might benefit.

Conclusion

This chapter has provided a brief overview of the rationale, methods and issues surrounding evidence-based practice. For many in primary care the message of evidence-based practice is neither new nor surprising. Good practitioners have always sought to keep their practice up-to-date. The processes of clinical governance should help all in primary care in their application of evidence-based practice.

Practical points

- Evidence-based practice is not new.
- It concerns the use of current best evidence in the care of individual patients.
- There are vast amounts of published research, not all of which is of good quality.
- Evidence-based practice provides a structured approach to finding, appraising and applying best evidence.
- There are useful sources of summarised research evidence for busy practitioners.
- The help of a good librarian can be invaluable.
- Primary care teams should have access to the internet and the Cochrane Library.
- Patients are increasingly better informed and practitioners need to be able to discuss the evidence with them.

References

1   Sackett DL, Rosenberg WMC, Gray JAM *et al.* (1996) Evidence based medicine: what it is and what it isn't. *BMJ.* **312**: 71–2.

2   Sacket DL, Richardson WS, Rosenberg W *et al.* (1997) *Evidence Based Medicine.* Churchill Livingstone, Edinburgh.

3   Chalmers I and Altman DG (eds) (1995) *Systematic Reviews.* BMJ Publishing, London.

4   Muir Gray JA (1997) *Evidence Based Healthcare: how to make health policy and management decisions.* Churchill Livingstone, Edinburgh.

5   Gill P, Dowell AC, Neal RP *et al.* (1996) Evidence based general practice: a retrospective study of interventions in our training practice. *BMJ.* **312**: 819–21.

CHAPTER FIVE

Disseminating and implementing evidence-based practice

Martin Eccles and Jeremy Grimshaw

This chapter analyses the effectiveness of a range of interventions which are used to bring about changes in clinical behaviour. No single intervention is effective under all circumstances. Multifaceted approaches are more likely to succeed.

Introduction

In all healthcare systems there is an increasing awareness of the need for quality assurance because:

- the resources available for healthcare are limited
- the variations in clinical practice are unexplained by characteristics of patients, their illnesses or the setting of care
- there is evidence of unacceptable standards of practice
- there is a lag between the emergence of research evidence and its incorporation into routine practice.

All of this is set against a background of demand for increasing professional and managerial accountability.

In response professional bodies have emphasised professionals' responsibilities to ensure quality of care, e.g. Royal College of General Practitioners,[1] and have issued guidelines, e.g. Royal College of Radiologists.[2,3] In addition, a range of policy initiatives has encouraged and supported quality assurance activities, for example the introduction of clinical audit,[4] the clinical effectiveness initiative[5] and the NHS R&D Programme.[6] The latest of these policy initiatives is clinical governance.[7]

Clinical governance is described as 'A new initiative' which includes 'action to ensure, *good practice is rapidly disseminated and systems are in place to ensure continuous improvements in clinical care*'[7] (our italics). If the clinical effectiveness element of clinical governance is to achieve its potential, and quality assurance and implementation activities are to be effective in improving the care that patients receive, there are two key steps: first, the rapid identification of effective treatments and healthcare interventions; and, second, the use of effective dissemination and implementation strategies to ensure the adoption of these effective interventions into routine practice.[8]

Identifying effective treatments and healthcare interventions

Over 20 000 medical journals are published each year containing research papers of variable quality and relevance. Yet the average time that a NHS consultant has available to read is about one hour a week. It is clearly impossible for healthcare professionals to keep up-to-date with primary research. To overcome this problem Guyatt and Rennie suggest 'that resolving a clinical problem begins with a search for a valid overview or practice guideline as the most efficient method of deciding on the best patient care'. [9] The issues of locating evidence are covered in Chapter 4. However, a number of points are worth emphasising here.

First, the best starting place for looking for systematic reviews is the Cochrane Library (Cochrane Collaboration, 1999). This contains:

- the Cochrane Database of Systematic Reviews, which currently includes 492 protocols and 522 systematic reviews undertaken by members of collaboration
- the Cochrane Controlled Trials Register, which currently includes over 200 000 trials
- the Database of Abstracts of Reviews of Effectiveness (DARE)
- the Cochrane Review Methodology Database.

Together these represent the most comprehensive starting place for searching for clinical trials and high-quality systematic reviews.[10]

Second, finding high-quality clinical guidelines can be problematic. Guidelines are published in the 'grey' literature, and are not indexed in the commonly available bibliographic databases (although there are a number of databases that specialise in 'grey' literature). For example, none of the guidelines published by the Agency for Health Care Policy and Research (AHCPR) can be found on Medline. Even when guidelines are published in indexed journals, the best search strategies have yet to be developed. In the Ovid version of Medline, practice guidelines can be identified under a variety of headings including: *guideline* (publication type), *practice guideline* (publication type), *practice guidelines* (MeSH heading), *Consensus Development Conference* (publication type) and *Consensus Development Conference, NIH* (publication type). A preliminary examination across several clinical areas suggests that *guideline* (publication type) is probably the most sensitive and specific single search term.

Fortunately, there are other resources available to help practitioners. In particular there are a number of sites on the internet which catalogue clinical guidelines (for example the AHCPR Guidelines Clearing House http://www.guideline.gov/). Full-text versions or abstracts of guidelines are available from some sites, and it is likely that these sites will become the best sources of guidelines in the future. Another strategy that primary care teams might consider is to develop a practice library of valid clinical guidelines, by appraising any guidelines they are sent.

Evidence-based implementation

Evidence is not self-implementing, and we now understand that active implementation strategies are required if new evidence is to be routinely incorporated into practice. However, most of the approaches to changing clinical practice are more often based on beliefs than on scientific evidence. This leads to the proposition that evidence-based practice 'should be complemented by evidence based implementation'. [11]

Systematic reviews of rigorous evaluations of different dissemination and implementation strategies (*see* Box 5.1) provide the best evidence for policy decisions about

---

Box 5.1:   Behaviour change strategies

Broad strategies
- continuing medical education
- clinical guidelines

Targeting specific behaviours
- preventive care
- prescribing
- referrals
- test ordering

Specific interventions
- dissemination of educational materials
- educational outreach visits
- local opinion leaders
- audit and feedback
- reminder systems
- computerisation

activities that promote clinicians' behaviour change. The Cochrane Effective Practice and Organisation of Care (EPOC) group undertakes systematic reviews of behavioural/professional educational, organisational, financial and regulatory interventions to improve professional practice and the delivery of effective healthcare services.[12] The EPOC editorial group has produced an overview of 44 systematic reviews of behaviour change strategies,[13] a summary of which is presented here.

Broad strategies

The group found 15 reviews focusing on broad strategies (involving a variety of strategies targeting a variety of behaviours) including: continuing medical education (CME), dissemination and implementation of guidelines, and other programmes to enhance the quality and economy of primary care.

Continuing medical education

Davis and colleagues have carried out a series of reviews of CME, the latest of which was published in 1995.[14] In that they identified 99 studies involving 160 comparisons of CME interventions. Improvements in at least one major endpoint were identified in 68% of the studies. Single interventions likely to be effective included educational outreach, opinion leaders, patient-mediated interventions and reminders. These are described later in this chapter. Multifaceted interventions, and those interventions where the potential barriers were assessed in advance, were more likely to be successful.

The introduction of clinical guidelines

A review of passive dissemination of consensus recommendations concluded that there was little evidence that it alone resulted in behaviour change.[15] A later review of factors influencing compliance with guideline recommendations found that compliance was lower for recommendations that were more complex and less trialable.[16] In 1994 the Effective Health Care Bulletin reviewed studies evaluating the introduction of guidelines.[17] In 81 of 89 studies improved compliance with guideline recommendations was reported, and improvements in patient outcome were seen in 12 of 17 studies that measured outcome. The bulletin authors concluded that guidelines can change clinical practice. Guidelines were more likely to be effective if they took account of local circumstances, were disseminated by active educational interventions and were implemented by patient-specific reminders. There was inconclusive evidence about whether guidelines developed by the 'end users' (local guidelines) were more likely to be effective than guidelines developed without their involvement (national guidelines).

In another review of 102 studies of interventions to improve the delivery of healthcare services, it was observed that dissemination on its own resulted in little or no change in behaviour.[18] Furthermore, more complex interventions, whilst frequently effective, usually produced only moderate effects. The authors concluded that there are 'no magic bullets' for clinical behaviour change. There is a range of interventions that can lead to change, but no single intervention is always effective.

Similarly a review of the effectiveness of introducing guidelines in primary care settings identified 61 studies, which showed considerable variation in the effectiveness of a range of interventions.[19] Multifaceted approaches combining more than one intervention are more likely to be effective, but may be more expensive.

Outside of medicine the evidence on the effectiveness of implementation strategies is scarce. One review of studies evaluating the introduction of guidelines for professions allied to medicine (PAMS) found only 18 studies of generally poor quality.[20] There was insufficient evidence to determine the effectiveness of different strategies, although a number of studies suggested that guidelines could be used to support the extension of nursing roles.

In summary, there are examples of programmes that have been successful in improving aspects of primary care. But there remain significant gaps in our knowledge about what works best.[21]

Interventions to improve specific behaviours

Other reviews have focused on interventions that target specific behaviours, for example preventive care, prescribing, referrals, test ordering.

Preventive care

A number of reviews have examined a range of the interventions used to influence all aspects of prevention. One study found improvements in the process of care in 28 of 32 studies.[22] Significant improvements in the outcome of care, however, were present in only four of the 13 studies that measured outcome. In primary care a range of effective interventions has been identified, with multifaceted interventions including reminders coming out as the most effective.[23] Such interventions, however, may incur greater cost, and they need to be focused rather than a shotgun approach.[24]

Prescribing

To improve prescribing, mailed educational materials alone are generally ineffective.[25] Educational outreach approaches and ongoing feedback are usually effective, but there is insufficient evidence to determine the effectiveness of reminder systems and group education. Incidentally, Soumerai and colleagues, who carried out the review on pre-scribing,[25] also observed that poorly controlled studies were more likely to report sig-nificant results compared with adequately controlled studies! This emphasises the need for rigorous evaluation of dissemination and implementation strategies.

Other behaviours

We have reviewed interventions to improve outpatient referrals, but only found four studies that showed mixed effects.[26] It was difficult to draw any firm conclusions on the basis of the review. In a review of studies of interventions to modify test-ordering behaviour, 15 of 21 studies targeting a single behavioural factor were successful.[27] How-ever, only two of 28 studies targeting more than one behavioural factor were successful. It seems that multifaceted interventions that target one behavioural factor are more likely to be effective.

Specific interventions

Some reviews have focused on the effectiveness of specific interventions, as opposed to broad strategies (*see* Box 5.1).

Dissemination of educational materials

Freemantle and colleagues reviewed 11 studies evaluating the effects of disseminating educational materials (defined as the 'distribution of published or printed recommend-ations for clinical care, including clinical practice guidelines, audio-visual materials and electronic publications'. The materials may have been delivered personally or through personal or mass mailings). None of the studies found statistically significant improve-ments in practice.[28]

Educational outreach visits

Thomson and colleagues[29] reviewed the effectiveness of educational outreach visits defined as

> *The use of a trained person who meets with providers in their practice settings to provide information with the intent of changing the provider's performance. The information given may include feedback on the provider's performance.*

They identified 18 studies mainly targeting prescribing behaviour. The majority of studies observed statistical improvements in care (especially when social marketing techniques were used) although the effects were small to moderate. Educational outreach was observed to be more effective than audit and feedback in one study. It is not clear whether educational outreach is cost-effective.

Local opinion leaders

The same group reviewed the effectiveness of local opinion leaders defined as

The use of providers explicitly identified by their colleagues as 'educationally influential'.

They found improvements in at least one element of the process of care in six of eight studies, although these results were only statistically and clinically important in two of the trials.[30] In only one trial was there an improvement in patient outcome that was of practical importance. Nevertheless, local opinion leaders were observed to be more effective than audit and feedback in one study. It was concluded that using local opinion leaders resulted in mixed effects. Further research is required before the widespread use of this intervention could be recommended.

Audit and feedback

One review found that feedback was less effective than reminders for reducing the use of diagnostic tests.[31] Balas and colleagues,[32] reviewing 12 evaluations of physician profiling defined as *peer-comparison feedback*, discovered ten studies showing statistically significant improvements, but the effects were small. They concluded that peer comparison alone is unlikely to result in substantial quality improvement or cost-control, and may be inefficient. In Thomson and colleagues' review,[33] audit and feedback was defined as:

Any summary of clinical performance over a specified period of time. Summarised information may include the average number of diagnostic tests ordered, the average cost per test or per patient, the average number of prescriptions written, the proportion of times a desired clinical action was taken, etc. The summary may also include recommendations for clinical care. The information may be given in a written or verbal format.

Thirteen studies were found which compared audit and feedback to a no intervention control group.[33] Eight reported statistically significant changes in favour of the experimental group in at least one major outcome measure, but again the effects were small to moderate. The review concluded that 'audit and feedback can be effective in improving performance, in particular for prescribing and test ordering, although the effects are small to moderate'. The widespread use of audit and feedback was not supported by the review.

Reminders (manual or computerised)

The effectiveness of computer-based decision support systems (CDSS) has also been examined. Significant improvements were observed in: six of 15 drug dosing studies; one of five studies on diagnosis; 14 of 19 studies on prevention; 19 of 26 studies on general management of a problem; and four of seven studies measuring patient outcome. It was concluded that CDSSs may enhance clinical performance for most aspects of care, but *not* diagnosis.[34]

Computerisation

There have been two broader reviews of the effects of computerised systems,[35,36] in one case covering 30 studies on the effects of computers on primary care consultations.[35] It was observed that immunisation, other preventive tasks and some other aspects of performance improved. Consultation time, however, lengthened and there was a reduction in patient-initiated social contact. It seems that a range of different computer interventions improve care, including, provider prompts, patient prompts, computer-assisted patient education and computer-assisted treatment planners.[36]

Other interventions

There have also been reviews of other types of intervention, for example the effects of mass media campaigns on health services utilisation, where statistical improvements were seen in seven of 17 studies and meta-analysis suggested that campaigns do have an effect.[37] In a systematic review of continuous quality improvement (CQI) programmes, 43 single-site studies (41 used an uncontrolled before and after design) and 13 multisite (12 of which used a cross-sectional or uncontrolled before and after design) were examined.[38] The results from the uncontrolled before and after or cross-sectional studies suggested that CQI was effective, whereas all the randomised studies showed no effect. The predominance of single-site study designs made it difficult to attribute the observed effects to CQI.

Implications for policy and practice

Rigorous evaluations provide the best evidence about the effectiveness of different behavioural change strategies, and there are a number of consistent findings from evaluations to date. There are no 'magic bullets'.[18] Most interventions are effective under some circumstances; none is effective under all circumstances (*see* Box 5.2). Passive dissemination (e.g. mailing educational materials to targeted clinicians) and didactic

---

Box 5.2:   Interventions most likely to produce clinical behaviour change

- guidelines that take account of local circumstances
- guidelines disseminated as part of an educational programme
- educational outreach visits
- audit and feedback
- reminder systems
- multifaceted interventions focused on barriers to change

No single intervention is effective under all circumstances.

---

educational sessions are generally ineffective and unlikely to result in behaviour change when used alone. These approaches, however, may be useful for raising awareness of the desired behaviour change (*see* Box 5.3). Audit and feedback may be effective (especially for prescribing and test ordering), however, the effects are small to modest. Educational outreach is generally effective in changing prescribing behaviour, although most of the studies have been conducted in North American settings. There are a number of current trials which will provide evidence about the effectiveness of this approach in the UK. Reminder systems are generally effective for a range of behaviours. Multifaceted interventions targeting the various barriers to change are more likely to be effective than single interventions. Interventions based on an assessment of potential barriers are more likely to be effective.

Box 5.3   Interventions less likely to produce clinical behaviour change

- single interventions (rather than multifaceted)
- passive dissemination
- didactic lectures

Lectures may be useful for raising awareness.

Choosing implementation strategies

It is possible to choose a potentially successful strategy in the light of knowledge of the effectiveness of the interventions and knowledge of local barriers to implementing evidence-based practice. The information on barriers can be gleaned from interviews with individual patients or clinicians, group interviews or direct observation. For example, educational approaches (seminars and workshops) may be useful where barriers relate to healthcare professionals' knowledge. Audit and feedback may be useful when health-care professionals are unaware of sub-optimal practice. Social influence approaches (processes which encourage local consensus, educational outreach, opinion leaders, marketing, etc.) may be useful when barriers relate to the existing culture, routines and practices of healthcare professionals. Reminders and patient-mediated interventions may be useful when healthcare professionals have problems processing information within consultations. The presence of organisational barriers will require other sorts of specific interventions.

Conclusions

Clinical governance will require collaboration between clinicians and managers, who will need access to sources of high-quality evidence. Guidelines and systematic reviews provide the best source of evidence of the effectiveness of healthcare interventions. Reviews of the effectiveness of implementation strategies confirm that active dissemination and implementation of guidelines is required to ensure that the potential changes in practice occur. There is a variety of evidence-based implementation strategies, each of which is effective under certain conditions.

The choice of strategy should be based on a consideration of:

- which focused activities should be targeted
- at which specific healthcare professionals
- to overcome which perceived barriers to change.

Attention should also be given to likely available resources and the processes needed to manage change.

Practical points

- Evidence-based practice needs to be complemented by evidence-based implementation.
- Passive dissemination on its own does not result in behaviour change.
- No single intervention is effective in all circumstances – there are no 'magic bullets'.
- Multifaceted strategies, particularly those incorporating educational outreach, audit and feedback, and patient-specific reminders, are more likely to be effective.
- It is not known whether locally developed guidelines are more effective than national ones – they do need to take account of the local circumstances.
- It is more difficult to bring about complex behaviour change than simple or single change.
- Interventions that address perceived barriers to change are more likely to be effective.

References

1 Royal College of General Practitioners (1985) *Quality in General Practice. Policy Statement 2.* Royal College of General Practitioners, London.

2 Royal College of Radiologists (1995) *Making the Best Use of a Department of Clinical Radiology: guidelines for doctors* (3e). Royal College of Radiologists, London.

3 Petrie JC, Grimshaw JM and Bryson A (1995) The Scottish Intercollegiate Guidelines Network initiative: getting validated guidelines into local practice. *Health Bulletin (Edinburgh).* **53**: 345–8.

4 Secretaries of State for Social Services, Wales, Northern Ireland and Scotland (1989) *Working for Patients.* HMSO, London.

5 NHS Executive (1997) *Clinical Effectiveness Resource Pack.* Department of Health, Leeds.

6 NHS Executive (1996) *Research and Development. Towards an Evidence-based Health Service.* Department of Health, Leeds.

7 Department of Health (1997) *The New NHS: modern, dependable.* Cm 3807. The Stationery Office, London.

8 Eccles M and Grimshaw J (1995) Whither quality assurance? A view from the United Kingdom. *European Journal of General Practice.* **1**: 8–10.

9 Guyatt G and Rennie D (1993) Users' guides to the medical literature. *JAMA.* **270**: 2096–7.

10 Egger M and Smith GD (1998) Bias in location and selection of studies. *BMJ.* **316**: 61–6.

11 Grol R (1997) Beliefs and evidence in changing clinical practice. *BMJ.* **315**: 418–21.

12 Bero L, Grilli R, Grimshaw JM, Mowatt G and Oxman AD (eds) (1999) Cochrane Effective Professional and Organisation of Care Group. In: *The Cochrane Library*, Issue 4. Update Software, Oxford.

13 Effective Health Care Bulletin (1999) *Getting evidence into practice.* Bulletin no. 5. Royal Society of Medicine Press, London (also available from: http://www.york.ac.uk/inst/crd/ehc51.pdf).

14 Davis DA, Thomson MA, Oxman AD and Haynes RB (1995) Changing physician performance: a systematic review of the effect of continuing medical education strategies. *JAMA.* **274**: 700–5.

15 Lomas J (1991) Words without action? The production, dissemination, and impact of consensus recommendations. *Annual Review of Public Health.* **12**: 41–65.

16 Grilli R and Lomas J (1994) Evaluating the message: the relationship between compliance rate and the subject of practice guideline. *Medical Care.* **32**: 202–13.

17 Effective Health Care Bulletin (1994) *Implementing clinical guidelines. Can guidelines be used to improve clinical practice?* Bulletin no. 8. University of Leeds, Leeds.

18 Oxman AD, Thomson MA, Davis DA and Haynes B (1995) No magic bullets: a systematic review of 102 trials of interventions to improve professional practice. *Canadian Medical Association Journal.* **153**: 1423–31.

19   Wensing M, van der Weijden T and Grol R (1998) Implementing guidelines and innovations in general practice: which interventions are effective? *British Journal of General Practice.* **48**: 991–7.

20   Thomas L, Cullum N, McColl E, Rousseau N, Soutter J and Steen N (1999) Clinical guidelines in nursing, midwifery and other professions allied to medicine (Cochrane Review). In: *The Cochrane Library*, Issue 1. Update Software, Oxford.

21   Yano EM, Fink A, Hirsch SH, Robbins AS and Rubenstein LV (1995) Helping practices reach primary care goals. Lessons from the literature. *Archives of Internal Medicine.* **155**: 1146–56.

22   Lomas J and Haynes B (1988) A taxonomy and critical review of tested strategies of the application of clinical practice recommendations: from 'official' to 'individual' clinical policy. *American Journal of Preventive Medicine.* **2**: 77–94.

23   Hulscher M (1998) Implementing prevention in general practice: a study on cardiovascular disease. PhD thesis, University of Nijmegen, Nijmegen.

24   Snell JL and Buck EL (1996) Increasing cancer screening: a meta-analysis. *Preventative Medicine.* **25**: 702–7.

25   Soumerai SB, McLaughlin TJ and Avorn J (1989) Improving drug prescribing in primary care: a critical analysis of the experimental literature. *The Milbank Quarterly.* **67**: 268–317.

26   Grimshaw JM (1998) Evaluation of four quality assurance initiatives to improve out-patient referrals from general practice to hospital. PhD thesis, University of Aberdeen, Aberdeen.

27   Solomon DH, Hashimoto H, Daltroy L and Liang MH (1998) Techniques to improve physician's use of diagnostic tests. *JAMA.* **280**: 2020–7.

28   Freemantle N, Harvey EL, Wolf F, Grimshaw JM, Grilli R and Bero LA (1996) Printed educational materials to improve the behaviour of health care professionals and patient outcome (Cochrane Review). In: *The Cochrane Library*, Issue 4. Update Software, Oxford.

29   Thomson MA, Oxman AD, Davis DA, Haynes RB, Freemantle N and Harvey EL (1997) Outreach visits to improve health professional practice and health care outcomes (Cochrane Review). In: *The Cochrane Library*, Issue 3. Update Software, Oxford.

30   Davis DA, Haynes RB, Freemantle N and Harvey EL (1999) Local opinion leaders to improve health professional practice and health care outcome (Cochrane Review). In: *The Cochrane Library*, Issue 1. Update Software, Oxford.

31   Buntinx F, Winkens R, Grol R and Knotternerus JA (1993) Influencing diagnostic and preventative performance in ambulatory care by feedback and reminders. A review. *Family Practice.* **10**: 219–28.

32   Balas EA, Boren SA, Brown GD, Ewigman BG, Mitchell JA and Perkoff GT (1996) Effect of physician profiling on utilisation. *Journal of General Internal Medicine.* **11**: 584–90.

33   Thomson MA, Oxman AD, Davis DA, Haynes RB, Freemantle N and Harvey EL (1998) Audit and feedback to improve health professional practice and health care outcomes. Part I (Cochrane Review). In: *The Cochrane Library*, Issue 1. Update Software, Oxford.

34   Hunt DL, Haynes RB, Hanna SE and Smith K (1998) Effects of computer-based clinical decision support systems on physician performance and patient outcomes. A systematic review. *JAMA.* **280**: 1339–46.

35 Sullivan F and Mitchell E (1995) Has general practitioner computing made a difference to patient care? A systematic review of published reports. *BMJ*. **311**: 848–52.

36 Balas EA, Austin SM, Mitchell J, Ewigman BG, Bopp KD and Brown GD (1996) The clinical value of computerised information services. *Archives of Family Medicine*. **5**: 271–8.

37 Grill R, Freemantle N, Minozzi S, Domenighetti G and Finer D (1998) Impact of mass media on health services utilisation (Cochrane Review). In: *The Cochrane Library*, Issue 3. Update Software, Oxford.

38 Shortell SM, Bennett CL and Byck GR (1998) Assessing the impact of continuous quality improvement on clinical practice: what it will take to accelerate progress. *The Milbank Quarterly*. **76**: 1–37.

CHAPTER SIX

Quality improvement processes

Richard Baker and Mayur Lakhani

Quality improvement remains the core task of clinical governance. This chapter considers a framework for quality improvement processes in primary care. Whilst not presenting a complete model of clinical governance, quality improvement is discussed in relation to a more general model illustrated by examples.[1]

Introduction

Four elements must be in place for quality improvement to occur in primary care. The first is the creation of a culture (with its associated systems) that promotes interest in quality and facilitates quality improvement. The second requires the introduction of systems to identify obstacles to quality and quality improvement. The third involves developing strategies to overcome the particular obstacles so identified. Fourth, quality improvement should focus on known deficiencies in care, and appropriate changes monitored. Where improvements do not take place, further action will be required.

Quality systems in organisations

Basic principles

Clinical governance can be regarded as a type of quality system. Almost all moderate-sized commercial or industrial systems will have a quality system, the aim of which is to improve and maintain the quality of performance. The elements of quality systems vary

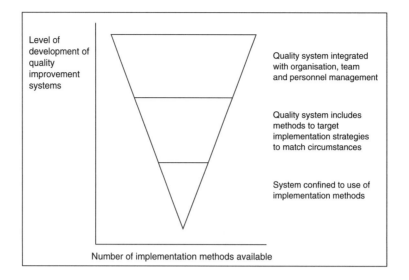

Level of development of quality improvement systems

Quality system integrated with organisation, team and personnel management

Quality system includes methods to target implementation strategies to match circumstances

System confined to use of implementation methods

Number of implementation methods available

Figure 6.1   The development of quality systems.

between different organisations, some organisations having more developed systems than others. The general process of developing a quality system is shown in Figure 6.1.

Typically, an organisation begins by utilising one method for establishing or improving quality. In the case of the health service, that method has been clinical audit. However, one method is rarely enough, because the number of problems encountered is usually more than can be solved by any single method alone. Thus, as time goes by, a wide range of methods comes into use. At some point, it becomes clear that the haphazard use of a variety of methods leads to much wasted effort and little impact. At this stage, the various methods must be brought together for a thorough review to take place.

One method may be identified as being particularly suited to solving one type of problem, whereas other methods are clearly not. Therefore, the next step in developing a quality system is to introduce mechanisms that identify specific problems and the appropriate methods necessary to solve them. Quality improvements should then take place. However, the pace of improvement slows down when it becomes clear that the final obstacle to change is the organisational culture itself.

If quality is to be guaranteed, the entire organisation needs to be constructed so as to ensure quality performance. This means that the quality system must become integrated with, and virtually indistinguishable from, the general management system.

Getting started in primary care groups

Dr Silvester had been appointed as the clinical governance lead to the Board of the recently established North Barchester Primary Care Group. Dr Silvester had been a member of the local Primary Care Audit Group and had been responsible for involving several local practices in audit. However, she recognised that there would be more to clinical governance than audit alone, but there was very little guidance about how clinical governance should be established or what it would consist of. Her role as clinical governance lead seemed both daunting and ill-defined.

It is possible to assess the level of development of the quality systems in place in primary care using Figure 6.1. In general, most primary care groups for instance, will have relatively poorly developed systems. There may be some audit undertaken, and a certain amount of education and training present. A complaints system will be in place. Thus, methods for quality improvement will be in use to varying degrees. The range of such methods will probably be limited, and they are unlikely to be integrated into systems for diagnosing significant quality problems and developing strategies to solve them.

The primary care group board is required to provide guidance for the introduction of clinical governance, a particular variety of quality system, to ensure that it gradually develops and becomes effective. The starting point is the creation of an appropriate culture, with practical systems for communication and decision-making. Quality of care depends ultimately on the performance of individuals. To perform at their best, individuals require the reward of job satisfaction, participation in making decisions about their work, support and understanding from the organisation for which they work, and the elimination of obstacles that prevent them performing to their best.

As Dr Silvester thought about the introduction of clinical governance into her primary care group in terms of quality systems in the commercial world, it became clear that the quality system in her group was at a very low level of development. It might take five years or longer fully to implement a reasonable system. She also recognised that it would be of limited value to concentrate her initial effort on merely increasing the range of improvement methods available. Simply promoting more audit and educational activities was not going to be enough. She needed to gain the support of her board for a long-term strategy to develop clinical governance in her primary care group.

The Board had already decided that the clinical governor needed to be clinically respected and to have the confidence of the practitioners within the primary care group. As Dr Silvester was a well-regarded member of the local audit group, the Board had decided to appoint her. Of particular importance were her highly developed interpersonal and communications skills. The Board felt that a confrontational and aggressive approach would be unlikely to succeed at a time when healthcare professionals were feeling particularly threatened by change and working under great difficulty and pressures.

The Board had particularly liked the approach recommended in the RCGP document, 'Practical guidance for clinical governors' which suggested treading a course between overoptimism and inactivity in the first year.[2] The Board was keen to ensure that primary healthcare professionals remained committed to quality improvement and therefore wished to adopt a supportive approach.

If the primary care group clinical governance system concentrated only on inspection, the consequence would be the demotivation of healthcare professionals. Such a bureaucratic approach would cause healthcare professionals to limit themselves to the bare minimum necessary to comply with clinical governance. In contrast, a culture that valued healthcare professionals, and balanced professional autonomy with accountability (without sacrificing the objective of detecting poor performance), would be more likely to lead to successful clinical governance. Dr Silvester and her board set aside a half-day meeting to discuss these issues and to agree their attitude towards clinical governance for the group.

In our example, the clinical governor and her board devoted the scarce resource of time to developing their ideas for clinical governance. This would be an appropriate first step for other groups, and having begun to develop ideas about clinical governance among those responsible for leading the group, the next step would be to develop a complementary culture within primary healthcare teams. Effective communication is the essential ingredient for developing a culture conducive to quality improvement, and the communication must be two-way, open, unimpeded and designed to generate trust. Face-to-face meetings are almost always necessary, but they should be supplemented by comprehensive and rapid written communication. One option would be to visit each primary healthcare team in turn for detailed discussions 'on their turf'. Another option is discussed in the next stage of the example.

Dr Silvester wrote to all primary healthcare teams and identified a clinical governance lead in each. She convened a meeting of the leads to discuss the opportunities for, and barriers to, clinical governance. As a result, the leads agreed a work plan for the next 12 months. They agreed to invite to their meetings the Primary Care Audit Group general manager and a GP educationalist from the local postgraduate department. The local leads identified a framework for developing clinical governance that included plans relevant to individual professionals, primary healthcare teams and the primary care group as a whole. A pertinent issue for the leads was to establish confidentiality and arrangements for data sharing within the primary care group and with the Board. The leads also planned a programme of team visits, by clinician peers, to develop an understanding of each team's philosophy, and its strengths and weaknesses.

The Board recognised that Dr Silvester could not deliver clinical governance alone. Her role was to offer leadership to ensure that the systems were in place and working and that she should be supported by the primary care group in the 'building of alliances to use existing skills and resources to maximum benefit'.[2] They also identified resources as a key issue and decided to convene a meeting with the health authority to discuss the possibility of protected time for teams to develop clinical governance. A policy for clinical governance for non-principals was also to be put in place. The group also decided to investigate mechanisms for helping sick doctors, and to sort out arrangements for an occupational health system for team members.

Identifying obstacles to change

Obstacles to quality improvement may arise within the primary care group itself, or within primary healthcare teams, or in relation to individual health professionals. Box 6.1 provides examples of obstacles to quality improvement.

Different approaches are needed to deal with different obstacles.[3] For example, if morale is low among members of a primary care group, and they feel unable to rise to the challenge of quality improvement, providing them with feedback from audit that shows their performance to be poor will do little to help. It could merely reinforce their belief that they are powerless to change things, and will depress morale even further. Instead, they need confident leadership that initiates small projects that are certain to succeed and as a result will enable self-confidence to grow.

It follows that a key first, and continuing, task for primary care group clinical governors is to identify the obstacles to change that must be faced, becoming attuned both to the mood of the primary care group and to the problems confronting the constituent teams and individuals. A variety of methods may be used to identify the obstacles to quality improvement and the levers for change that already exist in the primary care group. If employed effectively, the levers alone may be sufficient to promote

---

Box 6.1:   Examples of obstacles to quality improvements

Individuals

- lack of knowledge, skills or time
- poor personal health
- not aware of the need for change
- not convinced of the need for change

Teams

- poor communication about the change
- conflicting objectives
- lack of appropriately skilled personnel
- poor collaboration

Primary care groups

- limited resources
- low morale among members
- poor communication between healthcare teams
- lack of leadership
- low priority given to quality of care

the quality improvements that are needed. The methods for identifying obstacles and levers vary from informal communication to complex techniques such as focus groups or surveys of organisational culture.

Informal communication is always useful. If you do not understand why implementing improvement is proving difficult, go and ask the people involved; the answers are often revealing. However, there are some disadvantages to this approach. The respondents may not be representative, and they may not be able to identify the most important obstacles. Formal methods of investigation can allow a more complete description of the obstacles and levers, and can also enable them to be explored in greater depth. These methods cannot be discussed in detail here; a summary, with references, is found in Box 6.2. In choosing methods for identifying obstacles and levers, it should be remembered that information is needed about the primary care group as an organisation, the primary healthcare teams in the group, and individual professionals. One system for meeting these requirements is shown in Box 6.3.

Dr Silvester set up two schemes for identifying obstacles and levers. The first was used to detect problems in teamwork. She undertook a survey in which members of teams were asked to complete a brief questionnaire about their perceptions of teamwork. Individual responses were dealt with confidentially, but allowed her to identify the strengths and weaknesses of each team. Nine of the 12 teams appeared to be functioning satisfactorily, but three were in need of help.

Box 6.2:   Methods of identifying obstacles and levers

Individuals

- appraisal systems
- interviews
- questionnaires

Primary healthcare teams

- observation of team meetings
- visit by clinical governance lead to meet with leads of each team
- reports from team clinical governance leads
- questionnaires, e.g. the team diagnostic instrument[4]

Primary care group

- discussion by members of the board
- focus groups of members of the primary care groups[5]
- questionnaire about culture[6]
- questionnaire about teamwork[4]

Box 6.3: A strategy for identifying obstacles and levers in a primary care group

Individuals
Appraisal system introduced for all health professionals, with appraisal performed by clinical governance lead from neighbouring practices.

Teams
Visit by primary care group clinical governance lead to each practice to meet with teams.

Primary care group
Focus groups convened at intervals.

In one team the practice manager had been unwell and had lost a lot time from work. At the same time, the practice nurse had retired and a replacement had not been found. Dr Silvester asked the Board to provide emergency support, and a senior receptionist from another team was seconded to help with practice management and a locum practice nurse was found.

In the second team, there were difficulties with communication. Practice meetings were infrequent and members of the team were not involved in making plans. In consequence, the team was failing to respond to the changing demands of healthcare. In response, Dr Silvester arranged for a course organiser from a nearby vocational training scheme to facilitate practice meetings over a period of several months. As a result, the team was able to confront its problems in communication, work together to resolve them, and transform its approach to innovation and development.

The third team was a small, inner-city practice facing a heavy workload. The team was overwhelmed, unable to stand back and make plans for long-term development. Day-to-day pressures took precedence over everything else. Dr Silvester discussed these problems with her board and convinced it of the need for particular support through the provision of a salaried GP and a primary care nurse approved for prescribing. Over the course of the next year this additional support enabled the practice to devote more time to planning its future and taking control of its own destiny.

The second scheme was intended to support individual professionals in the primary care group. Dr Silvester set in place a personal development appraisal system for all GPs and nursing staff. The clinical governance leads in each primary healthcare team were invited to take on the role of appraising a team other than their own. The appraisals took place over a period of six months and as a result every clinician in the primary care group was able to discuss with a colleague their personal educational needs.

Monitoring performance

Since quality improvement activities cannot be relied upon to be successful, it is important to monitor progress. Clinical audit is the method by which performance can be monitored. Primary healthcare team professionals should by now have become familiar with clinical audit, and many detailed descriptions of audit are available.[7,8] However, since methodological weaknesses have been common in many audits undertaken in recent years, it is worth stressing a few points.

The first weakness in many audits is the limited use made of research evidence. The best current evidence should be used in selecting which aspects of care to assess. Clearly, there is little to be gained by expending effort in collecting data when it has not been established which aspects of care are truly important. In audit, review criteria are used to determine what information is needed (*see* Box 6.4 for definition), and time spent in clarifying the evidence to justify each criterion is time well spent. It is possible to reduce the time devoted to searching for evidence by drawing on good quality systematic reviews, guidelines or audit protocols developed by others.[9]

The second weakness common to many audits is in the use of samples. It is usually not necessary to select a sample of patients to be included in an audit, but when large numbers of patients are involved, and when good-quality computerised data are not available, it may be preferable to select a sample. Samples should be representative, and of sufficient size, to give confidence that the findings do reflect actual practice. Random samples are the safest method of ensuring representative results, and are easy to select. It is also simple to calculate a sample size, although all too often this step is omitted and in consequence the results of the data collection can be misleading. The methods to follow in calculating samples sizes and selecting random samples are described fully elsewhere.[7]

Box 6.4:   Terms used in audit and monitoring

Guidelines – systematically developed statements to assist practitioner and patient decisions about appropriate healthcare for specific clinical circumstances.[10]
Criteria – systematically developed statements that can be used to assess the appropriateness of specific healthcare decisions, services and outcomes.[10]
Audit protocol – a comprehensive set of criteria for a single clinical condition or aspect of organisation.[11]
Standard – the percentage of events that should comply with the criterion.[11]
Indicator – a measurable element of practice performance for which there is evidence or consensus that it can be used to assess the quality, and hence change in quality, of care provided.[12]

The third common problem is failure to complete the cycle. Of course, if performance is already satisfactory, a second data collection would be a waste of time, but usually this happy state of affairs is not the explanation for failure to complete the cycle. If computerised data are not readily available, a second data collection might require extra time and effort, but there is no other way to check that improvements have taken place. In the long term, primary care groups will need efficient data systems in order to make audit and the monitoring of performance a convenient routine.

Conclusion

The principal aim of clinical governance is to improve the quality of care provided to patients. This requires the creation of an appropriate culture, with systems that identify obstacles to quality improvement, removing such obstacles (or overcoming them when they cannot be removed) and monitoring performance through clinical audit. Where these core principles are implemented, primary care teams and groups should see improvements in the quality of the healthcare delivered. Equally, the health professionals within such teams and groups should find their working lives to be more enjoyable and fulfilling as a result.

Practical points

- Quality improvement is the core task of clinical governance.
- Experience from commerce and industry is helpful.
- A variety of quality improvement methods are needed.
- A supportive culture is essential.
- Clinical audit, good teamwork and clear communication play their part.

References

1   Baker R, Lakhani M, Fraser R and Cheater F (1999) A model for clinical governance in primary care groups. *BMJ*. **318**: 779–83.

2   Royal College of General Practitioners (1999) *Clinical Governance: practical advice for primary care in England and Wales*. RCGP, London.

3   Baker R, Hearnshaw H and Robertson N (1998) *Implementing Change with Clinical Audit*. John Wiley and Sons, Chichester.

4   Pritchard P and Pritchard J (1994) *Teamwork for Primary and Shared Care* (2e). Oxford Medical Publications, Oxford.

5   Krueger RA (1988) *Focus Groups. A Practical Guide for Applied Research*. Sage Publications, Newbury Park, CA.

6   Hearnshaw H, Reddish S, Carlyle D, Baker R and Robertson N (1998) Introducing a quality improvement programme to primary healthcare teams. *Quality in Health Care*. **7**: 200–8.

7   Fraser RC, Lakhani MK and Baker RH (eds) (1998) *Evidence-based Audit in General Practice. From Principles to Practice*. Butterworth-Heinemann, Oxford.

8   Crombie IK, Davies HTO, Abraham SCS and Florey C du V (1993) *The Audit Handbook. Improving Health Care Through Clinical Audit*. John Wiley and Sons, Chichester.

9   Fraser RC, Khunti K, Baker R and Lakhani M (1997) Effective audit in general practice: a method for systematically developing audit protocols containing evidence-based review criteria. *British Journal of General Practice*. **47**: 743–6.

10   Institute of Medicine (1992) In: MJ Field and KN Lohr (eds) *Guidelines for Clinical Practice: from development to use*. National Academy Press, Washington, DC, pp. 23–44.

11   Baker R and Fraser RC (1995) Development of review criteria: linking guidelines and assessment of quality. *BMJ*. **311**: 370–3.

12   Lawrence M and Olesen F for the Equip Working Party on Indicators (1997) Indicators of quality in health care. *European Journal of General Practice*. **3**: 103–8.

CHAPTER SEVEN

Appropriate use of data: the example of indicators

Richard Thomson

The ultimate criterion for the acceptance of a quality indicator is whether it leads to successful quality improvement projects

S Jencks[1]

The quality of primary care has many dimensions. This chapter reviews both the potential and limitations of quality/performance indicators, with illustrative examples from primary and secondary care. It provides a checklist of questions to ask when the use of indicators is being considered.

Introduction

If clinical governance is to support quality improvement in primary care, the issue of data quality is critical. This is not simply about technical properties, such as validity and reliability. The *quality of data use* is equally important, i.e. how data are collected, collated and fed back, who applies the data and the uses to which such data are put.

Although clinical governance incorporates monitoring and accountability, its main emphasis is on continuous quality improvement. There is a challenge, therefore, in reconciling monitoring, which implies a degree of judgement, with organisation-wide continuous quality improvement. Nowhere is this more evident than in the use of quality/perform-ance indicators.

What is a quality or performance indicator?

An indicator should be a rate, with both a numerator and a denominator. For example, the percentage of patients with diabetes who have had their cardiovascular risk status reviewed requires as a numerator the number of diabetic patients whose risk factors have been reviewed, and as a denominator the total number of diabetic patients. Further refinement of both the numerator and denominator allows more valid and reliable data collection, thus ensuring comparable data.

The Joint Commission on Accreditation of Health Care Organisations (JCAHO) defines an indicator as 'a quantitative measure that can be used to monitor and evaluate the quality of important governance, management, clinical, and support functions that affect patient outcomes'. Furthermore, 'an indicator is not a direct measure of quality. Rather, it is a tool that can be used to assess performance and that can direct attention to issues that may require more intense review'.[2] Indicators of performance aim to improve the quality of health services, ultimately resulting in improved patient care and popu-lation health.

However, indicators are but flags or screens; they are tools for generating further questions. Examination of an indicator begs the following questions. Why is this rate as it is? Why has it changed? Why does it differ from the rate in another practice or primary care group area? Such questions can only be answered by further exploration, preferably at a local level. Whilst indicator data can be collated centrally (and to support com-parisons they often need to be), the explanations for a local rate are local, as, more importantly, are the changes needed to improve quality. Thus, if primary care group A has a rate of generic prescribing well below that of other primary care groups, this merits local investigation, exploring such questions as: how does this vary across the primary care group, from practice to practice, or from GP to GP? Does this reflect a greater level of non-generic prescribing in certain British National Formulary chapters or drug types? What are the costs of non-generic prescribing? Where are the largest discrepancies (in terms of both prescription numbers and costs) worthy of exploration? When these questions are answered, more questions arise. For example, why are generic prescribing levels low in musculo-skeletal and joint diseases? What can we do to change this? Is there evidence to support policy or behaviour change? And so on (*see* Box 7.1 for an example).

Box 7.1:   Examples of effective use of indicators to improve quality in primary care

Prescribing ratio of inhaled steroids to bronchodilators in Lambeth, Southwark and Lewisham Health Authority

The health authority identified a range of primary care outcome measures, chosen on the basis of relevance to health, patient-centredness, application to broad populations, allowing comparison between providers, and attributable to primary care interventions. Practices received graphs of their rate compared with the authority mean. One example, the prescribing ratio of inhaled steroids to bronchodilators from PACT data, demonstrated approximately a fourfold variation across practices. The data were used as the focus for discussion during pharmaceutical advisor visits. The ratio also contributed to an index used to calculate practice prescribing budgets and to identify practices eligible for incentive payments towards more cost-effective prescribing. The local respiratory consultant, who had a special interest in primary care, made contact with practices where the prescribing ratio suggested that they might have the most to gain from specialist advice or outreach clinics.

Southampton and South-West Hampshire Health Authority primary care indicators

A wide range of indicators was developed, to be used in conjunction with information from PACT, the Family Health Services (FHS) Exeter system, the District Child Health system, practice annual reports and the local Health Care Purchasing system. A survey found that the majority of practices found the indicator set useful. However, the set was primarily used by the health authority's primary care group, and acted as a focus for pharmaceutical advisor and primary care medical advisor practice visits.

As an example, a practice with a high rate of inadequate cervical smears was identified and this finding was discussed at a subsequent practice visit. This process initiated further training of the practice nurses, with a marked reduction in the subsequent rate of inadequate smears.

One practice found a relatively low rate of infants being breast-fed at six weeks. This led to practice discussion, and review, which would not have happened in the absence of comparative data. A previously unidentified issue had been revealed by the indicator.

Source: McColl A, Roderick P and Gabbay J (1997) *Improving Health Outcomes: case studies on how English health authorities use population-based health outcome assessments*. Wessex Institute for Health Research and Development, Southampton.

Types and value of indicators

Indicators have been classified in a number of ways. The most common classification uses the Donabedian triad of structure, process and outcome, to which can be added access indicators, e.g. waiting times, and activity indicators, e.g. home visit rates. Alternatively, the Department of Health's Performance Assessment Framework lists six areas (see Box 7.2) providing a broad-based approach to assessing the performance of the NHS.[3]

Quality of care does vary, both between places (geographically) and over time (temporally). Whilst it may be possible to compare practice rates against published data (e.g. how does our primary care team's control of hypertension compare with published audits?), value is enhanced if there are contemporary data from comparable practice populations. A further potential benefit of comparison lies in the technique of benchmarking i.e. having identified other teams that appear to be performing better in hypertension control, can we learn from them? Whilst this implies being able to review others' rates, it can create concern about the inappropriate use of such comparisons. This worry can be overcome either through identifying voluntary benchmark partners (as hospitals do in the Performance Benchmarking Network), or through a system that uses anonymised data, but identifies and disseminates good practice.

Box 7.2:   The NHS Performance Assessment Framework[3]

Area	Example high-level indicator
Health improvement	Deaths from all circulatory diseases
Fair access	Adults registered with an NHS dentist
Effective delivery of appropriate care	Cost-effective prescribing
Efficiency	Generic prescribing
Patient/carer experience	First outpatient appointments for which patient did not attend
Health outcomes of NHS care	Emergency admission to hospital for those aged 75 and over

---

Technical characteristics of indicators

McColl and colleagues,[4] have stated that performance indicators for routine use by primary care groups should be:

- attributable to healthcare
- sensitive to change

- based on reliable and valid information
- precisely defined
- reflect important clinical areas
- include a variety of dimensions of care.

To this one could add measurable (quantifiable) and timely and, for indicators reflecting clinical treatment, evidence based. Unfortunately, an indicator that fully meets all these criteria does not exist. Rather, one has to consider the degree to which indicators meet these criteria, alongside other features. For example, an indicator could have good technical characteristics, but vary little from place to place, or reflect an area where change is difficult. All else being equal, these factors may limit its value in comparison with other, less technically sound, indicators. Furthermore, the use to which indicators will be put will also influence the relative importance of such criteria.

McColl and colleagues[4] describe an approach to link performance indicators to appropriate evidence-based interventions by:

- identifying interventions for which primary care has a key responsibility and which are of proven value, and
- estimating the potential burden of preventable deaths if the intervention is appropriately applied.

For example, influenza vaccination of all eligible patients aged over 65 in a population of 100 000 could prevent 146 deaths and 273 influenza episodes annually. If uptake was only 30%, 102 deaths and 191 influenza episodes could be prevented by full coverage. A primary care group could review comparative data on the percentage of the population vaccinated, and could feed the data back to primary care teams. This would enable them to compare their rate with others and to monitor change in uptake over time. A primary care group might then need to decide whether to address this area. What is the current local rate of uptake? How would the effort of creating change compare with, for example, increasing the use of aspirin after myocardial infarction or transient ischaemic attack? How best could the change be supported, e.g. targeting individual teams, incorporating it in continuing professional developmental programmes, local media campaigns, etc. (*see* Chapter 5)?

Campbell and colleagues[5] have developed an alternative approach, which combines appraisal of the literature with structured expert opinion, to develop relevant indicators (review criteria). A long list of potential indicators, garnered from review and appraisal of both the literature and guidelines in the areas of asthma, angina and diabetes, were considered by a consensus panel of experts. Two rounds of anonymous rating, for both necessity and appropriateness, with feedback to panellists of aggregate scores between rounds, were followed by face-to-face discussion. The emerging consensus was thus informed by the combined panel ratings and their variance. 'Strong scientific evidence' was present for only 26% of the potential indicators, which were rated as necessary aspects of care. Thus, if the development of indicators was based on randomised controlled trial evidence alone, a very limited number would have been generated, excluding many key elements of 'good' primary care practice. Many primary care interventions, such as the use of practice diabetic registers, could never be the subject of a randomised controlled trial.

The methods of McColl and Campbell offer potentially complementary approaches to developing relevant indicators for use in primary care. These are more likely to gain the approval of the professions, mainly because the development processes are seen as valid.

Data quality and accessibility

The use of indicators is highly dependent upon the quality of the underlying data source: data should be both complete and accurate. Thus, the rate of aspirin treatment in angina, based on disease-coded data, would require denominator data to be complete (all patients with angina have a diagnostic coding) and accurate (patients coded as having angina truly do have angina). Furthermore, production of these data from the information system should be straightforward.

Attribution to healthcare

Indicators may vary in their degree of attribution to primary care, and hence their relevance for primary care quality improvement. For example, the uptake of cervical screening is highly attributable to primary care (although of course patients may refuse), whereas the rate of emergency psychiatric admissions, an indicator proposed as a measure of the outcome of healthcare in the consultation preceding the NHS Performance Assessment Framework,[3] will depend partly upon primary care, but also on the relevant social services' provision and other factors.

Sensitivity to change

An indicator reflecting clinical practice should be sensitive to change. For example, decreasing the mortality from acute myocardial infarction is the goal of secondary prevention with aspirin, but monitoring this at a practice level using mortality is inappropriate. The numbers involved are too small, and monitoring changes in mortality will be insensitive to changes in the quality of care (*see* Box 7.3).

Box 7.3:   The capacity to detect real differences in quality

Mant and Hicks[14] considered the situation of a hospital admitting 450 patients per year to its coronary care unit with the diagnosis of myocardial infarction. The desire was to monitor the quality of care given over time. To detect a significant improvement in *outcome* (a reduction in mortality from 30 to 29%) with confidence, 73 years of data collection would be needed. In contrast, to confidently detect a significant improvement in a *process* of care (percentage of patients prescribed thrombolytic therapy), which would lead to an equivalent reduction in mortality from 30 to 29%, only four months of data collection would be required. The same issue is highlighted in comparisons between hospitals. The authors concluded that 'even with data aggregated over three years, with a perfect severity-adjustment system and identical case ascertainment and definition, disease specific mortality rates are an insensitive tool to compare the quality of care between hospitals'.

Reliable, valid and comprehensive

An indicator should measure what it seeks to measure (validity) and do so consistently (reliability). Validity is a complex concept. Suffice it to say that a measure is valid if:

- it is a potential marker for quality of primary care (face validity or relevance), and
- it measures what it purports to measure (for example a Read-coded stroke reflects a gold standard diagnosis of stroke).

An indicator is reliable if it is collected consistently in different places by different people at different times. This is highly dependent upon clear definitions and repeatable methods of data collection.

Campbell and colleagues undertook a national survey of potential indicators of primary care quality and identified 240.[6] These were then tested for face validity in a survey of managers and GPs. Only 36 of the indicators scored highly for validity, and the final list included no indicators for effective communication, care of acute illness, health outcomes or patient evaluation. Prescribing and gatekeeper indicators consistently received low validity ratings.

This is important because the quality of primary care has so many dimensions. Concentrating on the measurable may exclude important domains of quality. And even a set of indicators, as with the proposed primary care clinical effectiveness indicators, cannot at present cover all relevant domains. Indicators relevant to important dimensions, such as advocacy and consultation skills, would be very difficult to incorporate into any package. Nonetheless, a set of indicators should at least seek to address a range of relevant areas. The difficulty of this, in the light of Campbell's study, is clear.

How can indicator data support quality of care?

Internal or external use?

Anyone using or interpreting indicators to improve quality of care needs to be aware of their limitations, as well as their potential. This chapter includes examples from various sources, not all from primary care or from the UK. Nonetheless, they illustrate the key issues.

A fundamental decision is whether indicators will be used to make (external) judgements or to stimulate further investigation and quality improvement activity (from within), and, indeed, whether these different uses are compatible. Indicators could be used to make judgements. Is primary care team A better than team B? Is Dr Smith's prescribing of higher quality than Dr Jones's? This use is substantively different to feedback of anonymised comparative data to teams to support their own clinical audit or service development. Both approaches might be used in concert, but this is not without problems.[7-10] Reasons why external judgement on performance indicators may be inappropriate are:

* quality of primary care data
* choice of measure
* perverse incentives
* case-mix and context
* ability to distinguish
* chance.

Quality of primary care data

Whilst many practices are now computerised, and most use computers for prescribing (particularly repeat prescribing), computerised data are still limited. Few practices record diagnostic data, and, where they do, their completeness and accuracy vary. This problem, of missing and inaccurate data, has significant implications for both the selection and interpretation of indicators.

Even where data are more complete and accurate, such as Prescribing and Cost data (PACT), problems remain.[11] PACT data cannot be linked either to diagnoses, or to individual patients, to compare the appropriateness of prescribing at a diagnostic level. Equally, PACT data cannot be used to compare age- and sex-corrected prescribing adequately.

Developments in general practice computing and decision-support technology, may make future clinical data both more accessible and more complete for comparative analysis. For example, the PRODIGY system provides computerised guidelines with the potential to capture data relevant to clinical decisions on specific patients.

Choice of measure

Judgements imply ranking of practices. Not all the available measures might be used, and the indicators that are used will exclude important domains of quality (see above). Furthermore, the relative ranking of an organisation on the basis of performance indicators depends critically on which indicators are used (*see* Box 7.4).

Box 7.4:   Choice of indicator in coronary artery bypass surgery

Hartz and Kuhn[15] used a range of outcome measures and data sources (both clinical and administrative) from 17 US hospitals (with a total of 2687 coronary artery bypass surgery patients) to compare risk-adjusted rates. The correlations between adjusted hospital rankings, derived from either the clinical or the administrative databases, were not statistically significant for mortality, major complications or, indeed, for any complication. Whilst there was a reasonable correlation between risk-adjusted hospital rankings using the clinical database for mortality and major complications, the correlation between major complications and any complication was negative. These results not only suggested that assessing the quality of care by the use of administrative data may not be adequate, but, importantly, that quality assessment using clinical data may depend greatly on the outcome measure used. Thus, a hospital with a high ranking on the basis of one outcome measure may have a low ranking if other measures are used.

Perverse incentives

Indicator-based judgements may create perverse incentives. Participants will seek to do well on the chosen indicators. For example, the publicly available Patient's Charter indicators included the percentage of patients seen in accident and emergency units within five minutes. This sought to reflect the importance of immediacy of care to patients and, potentially, to patient outcome. However, accident and emergency departments appointed or redeployed 'triage' nurses, thereby producing improvements in the indicator, but not necessarily better care. Effective triage takes more than five minutes, so the response in many centres was simply to create the perjoratively titled 'hello nurse', there to greet but not to treat. Comparisons of performance against this indicator showed no correlation between the rating awarded and the use of either full triage or the length of triage.[12]

Some of the originally proposed primary care effectiveness indicators could have similarly perverse effects. An indicator on district nurse visits to the over-75s might lead to an inappropriate reduction in visits to the under-75s. This has been dropped from the NHS Performance Assessment Framework.[3] The ratio of inhaled corticosteroids and cromoglycate to inhaled bronchodilators could be increased by the indiscriminate prescription of steroid inhalers, with little improvement in patient care, and at increased cost. Comparing the rates of complaints might dissuade practices from seeking patient views. A practice with more complaints may have better systems for seeking patient views rather than poorer care.

Case-mix and context

Indicators are dependent on many factors beyond just the quality of care. Outcome measures, in particular, depend not only on the structures and processes of care, but also on patient characteristics such as age, sex, co-morbidity and socio-economic circumstances. A practice based in an area of socio-economic deprivation may thus appropriately have higher prescribing or admission rates.

An inadequate understanding of this can lead to quite erroneous judgements, which cannot be fully ameliorated by adjusting for case-mix, i.e. making allowances for the particular mix of population and conditions. It is not simply a matter of adjusting for extraneous factors to isolate variations that might be due to quality-of-care differences. Even with a high-quality, validated, case-mix adjustment system, problems can arise (*see* Box 7.5). Furthermore, the method of adjustment can affect ranking (*see* Box 7.6). Once again, judgements need to be made with extreme caution.

Ability to distinguish

We have already seen the difficulties that arise in demonstrating significant change in the quality of care where indicators cover only small numbers (*see* Box 7.3). This problem also impinges on the capacity to distinguish *between* providers on the basis of differences in indicators. Thus, there may be a real difference in quality of care but an inability to demonstrate it, i.e. the indicators chosen may not be sensitive enough.

The play of chance

Given the nature of health and healthcare, chance itself may lead to apparent differences between primary care teams or individual practitioners. This may lead to false denigration, i.e. things appear worse than they are in reality, or to false reassurance, i.e. things appear better than they are in reality.

Conclusions and lessons for primary care

The use of data to support clinical governance and quality improvement has been discussed with specific reference to quality or performance indicators. These have been the focus of considerably more debate since the publication of a *First Class Service*[13] and the NHS *Performance Assessment Framework*,[3] against a background of public concern following the Bristol case. This chapter has reviewed both the potential and the limitations of the use of such data in primary care. There are lessons to learn for primary care groups, from past experience in other sectors and other countries (particularly in

Box 7.5:   The New York State CABG register

The New York coronary artery bypass graft (CABG) register provides an example of a potential problem. This is a system of comparative, surgeon-specific, risk-adjusted CABG mortality rates which are made publicly available. The system uses a well-developed risk-adjustment process and good clinical data extracted by trained data collectors, with systems of data audit and quality control.[16–18]

Following its introduction it was noted that low-volume surgeons (those performing fewer operations) had consistently higher risk-adjusted mortality rates. Between 1989 and 1992, 27 low-volume surgeons (with a combined risk-adjusted mortality rate of 11.9% compared with a 3.1% statewide average) stopped performing CABG operations in New York State. In one hospital, the cardiac surgery programme had to be suspended until a new chief could be recruited and some hospitals reportedly assigned patients to selected surgeons.[17,18]

A case study from St Peter's Hospital, Albany, New York, showed how such data might be used beneficially.[19] This hospital had high risk-adjusted mortality, and decided to investigate further. They found that this was due not to higher-than-expected mortality amongst their low-risk patients, but to high rates of mortality among emergency cases. They felt that not enough time was devoted to stabilising patients. Following a restructuring of care, they saw marked improvements in the mortality rates in this sub-group, from a pre-intervention rate of 11 deaths among 42 emergencies in 1992, to a post-intervention period when none out of 52 died. This was achieved without the avoidance of high-risk patients, and demonstrates the importance of local audit, and subsequent change, in response to indicator data. It also shows that risk-adjusted data need careful interpretation. Overall, this hospital had a lower risk population of patients, but their higher apparent mortality was actually due to a problem with high-risk patients.

It is also reported that case-mix-adjusted mortality, in the state as a whole, fell over time following the introduction of the register, from 4.2% (1989) to 2.7% (1991).[20] However, a further analysis of the same data revealed that the recording rate for risk modifiers such as renal failure, congestive heart failure and unstable angina rose markedly over the same period.[21] For example, the rate of recorded renal failure rose from 0.4 to 2.8% and of chronic obstructive airways disease from 6.9 to 17.4%. This may reflect better recording of co-morbidity data as the system matured, but the size of change suggests another explanation, that of gaming, i.e. clinicians recording co-morbidities too. There is a perverse incentive on clinicians to record co-morbidities to 'upstage' the patients' risk and thereby show mortality rates in a better light.

Box 7.6:   Effect of risk-adjustment methods on ranking

Iezzoni and colleagues used 14 different severity adjustment methods in comparing mortality rates for pneumonia in 105 hospitals.[22] Whereas all the methods produced agreement on relative hospital performance more often than expected by chance, 30 hospitals were classified as outliers by one or more methods. The choice of method therefore, could have an important effect on the perceived performance of hospitals.

Box 7.7:   Relevant questions to ask of the use of data and indicators in primary care

- What are we seeking to achieve in the use of these data?
- Who will use the data? Will it be publicly available?
- Will the data be used to make judgements or to support clinical audit?
- Who will interpret the data?
- If judgements are to be made, how can we avoid or minimise the potential adverse effects of this approach?
- Will the data be anonymised or will primary care teams be identifiable?
- Where will the data come from? Is it readily accessible?
- What is the quality of the data source?
- Will we derive or collect our own data or use other readily available sources.
- Are the data items, and indicators derived from them, valid, reliable and sensitive to change?
- Are the definitions of data items clear and precisely defined?
- Do they reflect an important area of quality of care?
- Is this attributable to primary care?
- Is there evidence of important variation?
- Is the range of indicators reflective of the range of domains of quality in primary care?
- Are they based on evidence of effectiveness or consensus on good practice?
- Is there opportunity to create change?
- How will we engage local primary care teams and practitioners in the process?
- How will we support teams in the better use of such data?

---

secondary care). Equally, there is a growing awareness that these issues are generic regardless of the sector in which indicators are used.

Box 7.7 lists a series of questions and issues that primary care groups and primary care professionals, with a role in clinical governance, might ask themselves when considering the use of data and indicators. Box 7.8 lists sources of useful information and further reading.

Box 7.8:   Sources of useful information and further reading

Web sites

North West Thames Clinical Governance Site (includes examples of good practice, discussion documents)
http://www.doh.gov.uk/ntro/cgov.htm

National Primary Care Research and Development Centre (includes guidance on clinical governance and primary care indicators)
http://www.npcrdc.man.ac.uk/

Eli Lilly National Centre for Primary Care Audit
http://www.le.ac.uk/clinaudit/

National Centre for Clinical Audit
http://www.ncca.org.uk/

Norwegian Primary Care Indicators (home page of a Norwegian comparative indicator project in primary care)
http://www.uib.no/isf/sats/quality/httoc.htm

UK Quality Indicator Project (a UK-based project providing anonymised comparative feedback primarily for secondary and long-term care)
http://www.newcastle.ac.uk/~ndeph/webpage.html

Evidence-based medicine – primary care (Trish Greenhalgh)
http://www.ucl.ac.uk/primcare-popsci/uebpp/uebpp.htm#How

AHCPR Indicators CONQUEST database (a database of potential indicators with increasing links to the evidence base)
http://www.ahcpr.gov/qual/conquest.htm

The NHS Performance Assessment Framework
http://www.open.gov.uk/doh/coinh.htm

Further reading

Roland M, Holden J and Campbell S (1998) *Quality Assessment for General Practice: supporting clinical governance in PCGs.* National Primary Care Research and Development Centre. See: http://www.npcrdc.man.ac.uk/quality/quality.htm

Lally J and Thomson RG (1999) Is indicator use for quality improvement and performance measurement compatible? In: H Davies, M Tavakoli, M Malek and A Neilson (eds) *Managing Quality: strategic issues in healthcare management.* Ashgate Publishing, Aldershot, pp. 199–214.

Crombie, IK and Davies HTO (1998) Beyond health outcomes: the advantages of measuring process. *Journal of Evaluation in Clinical Practice.* **4**: 31–8.

Thomson RG, McElroy H *et al.* (1997) Maryland Hospital Quality Indicator project in the United Kingdom: an approach for promoting continuous quality improvement. *Quality in Health Care.* **6**: 49–55.

Practical points

- A quality or performance indicator should be a rate, with both a numerator and a denominator.
- As far as possible indicators should be: attributable to healthcare; precisely defined; based on complete, accurate, valid and reliable data; reflect important and evidence-based aspects of care; and be sensitive to change.
- Such indicators are not available for a number of important dimensions of good-quality primary care.
- Indicators may be used for external judgement and/or for internal quality improvement of an organisation, but different uses may have very different effects.
- Primary care can learn from experience in other sectors (particularly secondary care) and in other countries (particularly the USA).

References

1   Jencks SF (1994) HCFA's Health Care Quality Improvement Program and the Cooperative Cardiovascular Project. *Annals of Thoracic Surgery.* **58**: 1858–62.

2   Joint Commission on Accreditation of Health Care Organisations (1990) *Primer on Indicator Development and Application.* JCAHO, Chicago.

3   Department of Health (1999) *The NHS Performance Assessment Framework* (HSC 1999/ 078). Department of Health, London.

4   McColl A, Roderick P, Gabbay J, Smith H and Moore M (1998) Performance indicators for primary care groups: an evidence based approach. *BMJ.* **317**: 1354–60.

5   Campbell SM, Roland MO, Shekelle PG, Cantrill JA, Buetow SA and Cragg DK (1998) Development of review criteria for assessing the quality of management of stable angina, adult asthma, and non-insulin dependent diabetes mellitus in general practice. *Quality in Health Care.* **8**: 6–15.

6   Campbell SM, Roland MO, Quayle JA, Shekelle PG and Buetow S (1999) Quality indicators for general practice: which ones can general practitioners and health authority managers agree are important and how useful are they? *Journal of Public Health Medicine.* **20**(4): 414–21.

7   Davies HTO and Lampel J (1998) Trust in performance indicators? *Quality in Health Care.* **7**: 159–62.

8   Crombie IK and Davies HTO (1998) Beyond health outcomes: the advantages of measuring process. *Journal of Evaluation in Clinical Practice.* **4**: 31–8.

9   McKee M and Hunter D (1995) Mortality league tables: do they inform or mislead? *Quality in Health Care.* **4**: 5–12.

10   Thomson R and Lally J (1998) Clinical indicators: do we know what we're doing? *Quality in Health Care.* **7**: 122–3.

11   Majeed A, Evans N and Head P (1997) What can PACT tell us about prescribing in general practice? *BMJ.* **315**: 1515–19.

12   Edhouse JA and Wardrope J (1996) Do the national performance tables really indicate the performance of an accident and emergency department? *Journal of Accident and Emergency Medicine.* **13**: 123–6.

13   Department of Health (1998) *A First Class Service: quality in the NHS.* Health Service Circular: HSC (98)113. Department of Health, London.

14   Mant J and Hicks N (1995) Detecting differences in quality of care: the sensitivity of measures of process and outcome in treating acute myocardial infarction. *BMJ.* **311**: 793–6.

15   Hartz AJ and Kuhn EM (1994) Comparing hospitals that perform coronary artery bypass surgery: the effect of outcome measures and data sources. *American Journal of Public Health.* **84**: 1609–14.

16   Hannan EL, Kumar D, Racz M, Siu AL and Chassin MR (1994) New York State's cardiac surgery reporting system: four years later. *Annals of Thoracic Surgery.* **58**: 1852–7.

17   Hannan EL, Siu AL, Kumar D, Kilburn H and Chassin MR (1995) The decline in coronary artery bypass graft surgery mortality in New York State. *JAMA.* **273**: 209–13.

18   Chassin MR, Hannan EL and DeBuono BA (1996) Benefits and hazards of reporting medical outcomes publicly. *NEJM.* **334**: 394–8.

19   Dziuban SW, McIlduff JB, Miller SJ and Dal Col RH (1994) How a New York cardiac surgery program uses outcomes data. *Annals of Thoracic Surgery.* **58**: 1871–6.

20   Hannan EL, Kilburn HJ, Racz M, Shields E and Chassin MR (1994) Improving the outcomes of coronary artery bypass surgery in New York State. *JAMA.* **271**: 761–6.

21   Green J and Wintfeld N (1995) Assessing New York State's approach. *NEJM.* **332**: 1229–32.

22   Iezzoni LI, Schwartz M, Ash AS, Hughes JS, Daley J and Mackiernan YD (1996) Severity measurement methods and judging hospital death rates for pneumonia. *Medical Care.* **34**(1): 11–28.

CHAPTER EIGHT

Reducing risk in primary care

Peter Hill

The artistic sense of perfection in work is another much-to-be-desired quality to be cultivated. No matter how trifling the matter on hand, do it with a feeling that it demands the best that is in you, and when done look it over with a critical eye, not sparing a strict judgement of yourself.

Sir William Osler (1849–1919)[1]

This chapter explores the nature of clinical and non-clinical risk in primary care, and describes a systematic approach for assessing and reducing risk.

Introduction

The best defence against clinical risk in primary care is a consistently high standard of practice. The introduction of clinical governance is intended to address the well-documented variations in clinical care, and to avoid or prevent inappropriate care.[2] The identification, assessment and management of risk, therefore, should be welcomed, and not viewed negatively. Members of the general public understand the concept of risk, and apply it routinely to aspects of everyday life. In simple terms many adverse incidents can be foreseen and are entirely preventable; being purely reactive is just not good enough. A positive and proactive, systematic approach to managing both clinical and non-clinical risk is needed. The question is how?

First, scrutinise all the various activities carried out in a primary care setting. Then identify the possible risks, and grade them according to their potential frequency and severity. Try to eliminate those risks that can be eliminated, while mitigating the impact of those that cannot. And put into place mechanisms to absorb the likely consequences of the risks that still remain (*see* Box 8.1).[3]

Box 8.1:   Risk management

Risk management is a proactive approach which:

* *addresses* the various activities of an organisation
* *identifies* the risks that exist
* *assesses* those risks for potential frequency and severity
* *eliminates* the risks that can be eliminated
* *reduces* the effect of those that cannot be eliminated
* *puts into place* mechanisms to absorb the consequences of the risks that remain.

Perhaps, for the first time, clinical governance offers the opportunity to bring together the many strands that promote quality in clinical settings.[4] In hospitals, some systems are already in place, for example those for handling complaints, non-clinical risk management and clinical audit, but this may be less the case in primary care.[5]

Clinical risk in primary care

Clinical risk in primary care is often thought of in terms of the risk of litigation. Indeed there is growing awareness of an increasing resort by patients to legal processes, although there is no evidence of a decline in the quality of care. Litigation is therefore, and perhaps not surprisingly, the risk foremost in many practitioners' minds. This chapter is concerned with a broad approach to the issues of risk in primary care, and the reader is referred elsewhere for an introduction to litigation in medicine,[6] and for a detailed treatment of the subject.[7]

The nature of clinical risk can be best understood by considering it from the perspective of patients, practitioners (GPs and the other health professionals working as part of the primary care team) and procedures (or systems).

Patients

Certain groups of patients pose higher risks to the primary care team than others. For example, the question of blame is more likely to arise in cases involving children and young adults, especially if a death occurs, as this is now such a relatively rare event.

Foremost among these are young children, and the most obvious fear here is that of missing a diagnosis of serious illness, particularly meningitis. With children there can be difficulties in history taking, clinical examination, diagnosis and management. Of particular importance is the need to recognise the seriously ill child, and refer on, even when the complexity or rarity of the illness may reasonably defeat the most conscientious practitioner. Equally practitioners need to make special arrangements to review small children with acute illnesses, where there is a potential for the development (sometimes rapidly) of serious illness.

Practitioners and primary care teams

In considering clinical risk from the perspective of the practitioner, it is necessary to deem every dimension and aspect of clinical care as having the potential to be a problem. A risk can occur as a result of the failure of either an individual or a system. Patients have a right to good standards of clinical practice and care from their doctors and nurses.[8] Practitioners are expected to be professionally competent and perform consistently well.[9] In this they have always to strike a balance between the potential for doing good and the potential for doing harm – above all, perhaps, avoiding doing patients harm.

Increasingly, practitioners in primary care work together in primary care teams based on general practices of two or more doctors. All would like to work with 'perfect' colleagues (*see* Box 8.2).

Box 8.2:   Characteristics of the consummate colleague

The practitioner of today and tomorrow should be:

- providing comprehensive and continuing primary care
- clinically competent
- caring, compassionate and able to communicate
- well-organised and an efficient user of time
- able to delegate
- an effective administrator
- able to work in a team
- committed to audit and peer review
- committed to keeping up-to-date.

In primary care, the defining characteristic is that the practitioners provide personal, primary and continuing care to individuals and families. Such care inevitably spans the spectrum from preventive care and early diagnosis, through treatment, care, rehabilitation, palliative and terminal care, to bereavement and beyond. Thus the potential for risk is wide.

When patients are seen, they can reasonably expect that a suitable assessment of their condition will be made. This involves taking an adequate history and performing a competent clinical examination. Thereafter, they can expect relevant investigations, referral to specialists, or others, as necessary, and appropriate treatment and review.

This approach will be complemented by:

- good communication
- consent being sought appropriately
- the maintenance of confidentiality
- the keeping of clear and accurate contemporaneous records
- effective teamworking.

It is known, for example, that GPs who spend longer explaining things to the patient prescribe less.[10] In so doing they are exposing their patients to less risk of adverse drug reaction. (The same is likely to be true of nurse prescribers in the future.)

Whilst every step of the pathway has potential pitfalls, the practitioner or team should not be paralysed for fear of making a mistake. Patients and their carers should take comfort from the mechanisms assuring quality through clinical governance and revalidation.

Procedures and systems

A central ingredient in meeting these responsibilities is the extent to which the primary care team is easily accessible to patients. This includes being available for urgent consultations, and means having well-run systems for seeing patients during normal working hours and suitable arrangements out-of-hours.

It is easy to think of the administrative aspects of primary care as being of secondary importance to the all-important face-to-face contact with patients and their families. Consulting with patients remains the central task of healthcare, but should not diminish or override important aspects of management. The very notion of 'catching up with the paperwork' is not characteristic of an efficient and effective modern practitioner. Both doctors and nurses must now possess a wide range of ancillary skills and attributes, and should also have the benefit of good practice management. The patient is, after all, no less poorly served by a delayed referral or forgotten house call through administrative failure, than by poor clinical care.

It is worth noting that, in relation to the risks taken or problems incurred by members of the primary care team, the GP or practice partnership may be vicariously liable. That is they take on, or substitute for, the individual's responsibility. This is generally true for staff employed directly by the practice (secretaries and receptionists; practice-employed nurses), but may be less clear for other health professionals 'attached' to the practice. Health visitors, community nurses, midwives, chiropodists and physiotherapists will usually be covered by their employing organisation, normally an NHS trust.

The position with regard to locums employed by the doctor or practice is less clear. The locum may be employed by an agency or a deputising service, and all should carry their own insurance through a medical defence organisation. In any event, they are answerable to the GMC as a registered medical practitioner. On the other hand, under their Terms of Service GP principals are responsible for all the acts and omissions of those acting on their behalf.

Non-clinical risks

Risks relating to non-clinical issues account for almost a third of complaints notified to the Medical Defence Union.[11] Practice premises can present significant hazards for the unwary.* The Health and Safety at Work Act[12] requires any practice with five or more staff to have a health and safety policy, and practices should undertake an assessment of all health and safety risks, to patients, visitors and staff.

Obvious potential risks include fire, structural hazards, for example risks to children from stairs and stairwells (such as those with widely spaced bars) and ornamental ponds, and possible access to hazardous chemicals. From the staff perspective, suitable arrangements should be in place for the disposal of sharps (both handling on the premises and collection for destruction), biological materials and other waste. Appropriate and secure arrangements are required for drugs, especially scheduled drugs, medicines and chemicals, as well as pathological specimens.

The increasing risk of violence, or threats of violence, to NHS staff has been the subject of considerable media coverage, and of concern to patients and staff alike. Problems have been particularly evident in hospital accident and emergency departments (prompting NHS Executive advice on security[13]), but primary care staff are not immune. Procedures should be in place to protect all staff from the potential risk posed by the very small number of patients known to be dangerous. For instance, do staff know how to raise the alarm? Are there always two members of staff on duty together? Does the practice know where the doctors and nurses are doing their visits? All staff, including doctors, may need training in how to handle difficult or threatening telephone calls, and in techniques for coping with aggressive or violent behaviour.

While the preparation and handling of food is unlikely to be a major activity in most practices, legislatory requirements, common sense and good practice standards should be the norm. Basic hygiene principles should self-evidently be practised in organisations whose business is health. These should apply to staff kitchens, beverage and eating areas, food storage, as well as toilet and washing facilities. As with all protocols, guidelines and procedures, regular review and revision, if necessary, should be carried out.

---

* A hazard is a source of danger such as a sharp object or improperly maintained machine. A risk exists when there is exposure to the hazard and harm is possible.

Risk assessment

Some risks are obvious and easy to identify; others are not. Any approach to risk assessment, therefore, needs to be both detailed and systematic. One model, derived from industry, involves creating a matrix to relate potential risks or hazards to possible sources of risk.[3] (Having worked in a practice where the light bulbs, even in the reception area, disappeared mysteriously, and with monotonous regularity, I would not now under-estimate the capacity to be surprised by what can happen.) Box 8.3 shows how the matrix could be used in primary care.

Procedures (or practice systems) are a potential source of risk. They can be inherently flawed, and human beings make mistakes. Common problems include: failure to make a referral having agreed with the patient that this is an appropriate course of action; prescribing errors; lack of monitoring of patients with chronic diseases, particularly those on regular or long-term therapy; failure to act on abnormal test results; and failure of communication (*see* Box 8.4).

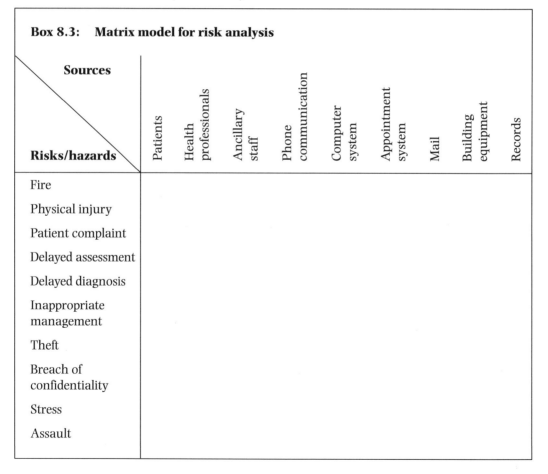

Box 8.3:   Matrix model for risk analysis

Risks/hazards \ Sources	Patients	Health professionals	Ancillary staff	Phone communication	Computer system	Appointment system	Mail	Building equipment	Records
Fire									
Physical injury									
Patient complaint									
Delayed assessment									
Delayed diagnosis									
Inappropriate management									
Theft									
Breach of confidentiality									
Stress									
Assault									

Box 8.4: Common problems with procedures or practice systems

Example of procedure or system at fault:

Possible remedies:

Delayed assessment of illness
- Arrangements for daily urgent appointments
- Protocol for accepting requests for home visits

Delayed referral
- Computerised or pre-printed proformas that include triggers for history, findings, medication, past medical history, family history, allergies, etc.
- Dictate or complete there and then (benefit of enhanced communication/greater patient confidence)
- Practice system with strict deadlines for turn-around of dictation, proof-reading, correcting, revising and signing

Acting on incoming information: outpatient or discharge letters, results of pathology, X-ray and other tests
- Systems for incoming mail, reports, etc., possibily including:
  - logging and dating
  - multiple-choice box stamps (for action, for info, see/ring patient, copy, file, etc.)
  - doctor to sign

Errors in prescribing
- Computerised systems
- Diligence
- Error trapping

Monitoring chronic illness
- Special clinics
- Guidelines and protocols
- Audit

Monitoring regular or long-term therapy
- Guidelines and protocols
- Defaults for review, e.g. 6 months or 1 year
- Audit

Communication between members of the primary care team
- Regular team meetings (formal and informal)
- Message books and proformas
- All use a single health record

Reducing the risks

The key elements in reducing risk include properly recruited and well-trained staff, clear procedures, regular monitoring and a safe environment. Donabedian has highlighted the relationship between the technical aspects of care, the interpersonal aspects and the environment in which healthcare is provided (*see* Figure 8.1).[14]

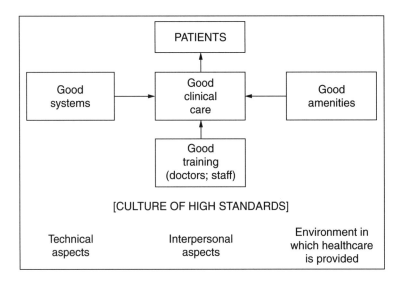

Figure 8.1   Good clinical care.

Properly recruited and well-trained staff

If the best defence against clinical risk in primary care is through a culture that promotes high standards of practice, then it follows that high-quality training underpins high-quality care. A clear commitment to training GPs, allied healthcare professionals and ancillary staff contributes much to the overall ethos of a primary care team. Indeed, being able to demonstrate high standards of clinical practice and appropriate clinical and administrative systems is a prerequisite for approval as a trainer in GP vocational training.[15] Similarly, student nurses gain immensely from being part of a supportive, reflective team where lifelong learning is encouraged.

Good training also needs to be complemented by good employment practice. The rigorous application of sound recruitment and selection procedures should eliminate (or at least minimise) the risk of appointment of unsatisfactory or unsuitable staff, be they doctors, other health professionals, or practice managerial or administrative support staff. Good practice in these fields includes detailed consideration of job purpose and description, person specification, checking registered qualifications and taking up of references (even for locum appointments), appropriate health checks, and preventive measures in line with current legislation and guidance. In particular, practices employing staff need to take account of equal opportunities, race discrimination and disability legislation. Proper recruitment needs to be followed by induction, (initial) supervision, where and as appropriate, and regular appraisal and performance review, with constructive feedback.

Clear procedures and good records

Although the evidence that good clinical records lead to good care is hard to find, good records can help support the demonstration of high standards of care and provide the basis for a robust defence if standards of care are questioned. Record-keeping systems extend to surgery and clinic attendances, to home visits and, increasingly, to telephone consultations, not least those involving nurse triage.

Even 'minor' illness may turn out to be major, and may only be judged as inconsequential in retrospect. All patient contacts should be recorded, and each entry should include, albeit briefly in the hurly-burly of practice, as appropriate:

- the date
- the patient's presenting complaint (using the patient's own words can be useful)
- clinical findings (positive and appropriate negative findings; systems examined)
- test results
- a diagnosis, diagnostic possibilities considered or even clinical impressions (including the patient's understanding of the problem)
- a management plan (arrangements for further investigation if necessary; treatment)
- arrangements for review (either planned or, if appropriate, what is to be done if things do not go according to plan).

Structured records help alert the healthcare worker, especially those who do not know the patient well. Even if the patient is well known, few of us can retain or recall accurately all salient features of their medical history without prompts and reminders. Information on important past medical and social history or life events, drug therapy, allergies and the present position on preventive measures such as blood pressure readings, or the most recent cervical smear and its result, should be readily available, not least to other members of the team.

Whilst computerised records can greatly facilitate all of this (e.g. with reminders of outstanding preventive measures), logically structured and systematised manual records can achieve the same through summary cards or special recording cards for particular categories of patient.

Because such information is important to have to hand for all consultations, and because home visits can represent the more serious end of the spectrum of illness, records (or at least a computer summary) should be available for home visits. Notwithstanding the practical and logistical difficulties this may pose at certain times (e.g. out of hours), this remains a good principle.

Safe environment

Patients expect information about them to be treated as confidential. There are exceptional circumstances where breaching this general principle may be appropriate, although advice should usually be sought in such cases. When considering issues relating to the disclosure of confidential information, it is easy to overlook the risk of inadvertent breaches of confidentiality. This is especially true of reception desks, for example, where personal and confidential details may easily be overheard. Background music can help reduce this risk.

Thought should be given to how the structure of the building can influence the protection of patient confidentiality. Many practices have a dedicated interview room or, at least, make available a suitable office for the purpose. All staff should be trained about the nature and fundamental importance of confidentiality and how to ensure it is maintained. Indeed, investment may be needed to improve the surgery premises in this regard. This may include the sound-proofing of doors and windows, especially in rooms where patients are interviewed. Each practice should nominate a lead person for confidentiality and security issues in line with the recommendations of the Caldicott Committee.[16]

Priority areas for action

First, high standards of thoughtful, clinical care are the bastion against risk and failure. Simply, this means doing the right things to the right people, and doing them right first time. Does the team have sufficiently robust systems of information to provide corroboration that the right things are being done and in the right way? Are the right people active in audit and reflection? Has the team undertaken an exercise to identify and assess risk?

Second, there must be the capacity to handle the workload effectively, through appropriate management, organisation and clinical leadership. No one model can be prescribed or is even desirable. Diversity remains one of the great strengths of primary care. But idiosyncratic approaches cannot be used as a smokescreen for poor standards of care. Who, for example, monitors the appointments system?

Third, is there a proper training programme for *all* staff? The NHS Human Resource Strategy has underscored the need for staff appraisal. By March 2000 it is intended that the majority of NHS staff will have personal development plans. Personal development planning (*see* Chapter 12) adopts a systematic approach to training and development. Who is responsible for ensuring that staff can do the job they are doing, as well as enabling them to meet their legitimate professional aspirations in the future? Is the team developing a Practice Professional Development Plan?

Fourth, does the team foster a 'no-blame' culture in which all are valued, and all can speak and be heard? For how else can the wisdom of a receptionist check or balance the folly of a senior partner?

Practical points

- Many adverse events can be foreseen and prevented.
- Risk management is a proactive and systematic approach to reducing risk and the impact of any risk which cannot be eliminated.
- In primary care risk should be considered from the perspective of patients, practitioners and procedures.
- A third of complaints to the Medical Defence Union concern risks relating to non-clinical issues.
- Risk needs to be assessed systematically.
- The best ways to reduce risk include properly recruited and well-trained staff, clear procedures and good records, and a safe environment.

Further reading

Partone – Communication (1998) *Risk Assessment for General Practice*. Medical Defence Union, London.

References

1   Osler W (1903) The master word in medicine. *Montreal Medical Journal.* Aequanimitas and other addresses.

2   Bloor K and Maynard A (1998) *Clinical Governance: clinician, heal thyself?* IHSM, York.

3   NHS Executive (1996) *Risk management in the NHS.* Department of Health, London.

4   Thomson R (1998) Quality to the fore in health policy – at last. *BMJ.* **317**: 95–6.

5   British Association of Medical Managers (1998) *Clinical Governance in the New NHS.* BAMM, Stockport.

6   Williams I (1995) Containing risk in general practice. In: C Vincent (ed) *Clinical Risk Management.* BMJ, London.

7   Scott W (1995) *The General Practitioner and The Law of Negligence.* Cavendish, London.

8   General Medical Council (1998) *Good Medical Practice.* GMC, London.

9   General Medical Council (1998) *Maintaining Good Medical Practice.* GMC, London.

10 Audit Commission (1994) *A Prescription for Improvement: towards more rational prescribing in general practice.* HMSO, London.

11 Lee R (1998) Risk management. In: D Garvie (ed) *The Members' Reference Book 1998/99.* Royal College of General Practitioners, London.

12 Health and Safety at Work Act 1974. HMSO, London.

13   North M, Bardsley A and Regan J (1997) *Effective Management of Security in A&E*. NHS
      Executive, London.

14   Donabedian A (1980) *The Definition of Quality and Approaches or its Assessment*. Health
      Administration Press, Ann Arbor, MI.

15   The Joint Committee on Postgraduate Training for General Practice (1998) *Recommen-
      dations to Deaneries on the Selection and Re-selection of General Practice Trainers*. JCPTGP,
      London.

16   Department of Health (1999) *Caldicott Guardians*. Health Services Circular: HSC(99)012.
      Department of Health, London.

CHAPTER NINE

Significant event auditing

Mike Pringle

> This chapter begins with two clinical cases, straightforward primary care cases, that illustrate the power of significant event auditing. Terms are then defined and the literature reviewed. Finally, the author describes his personal experience over more than a decade of regular significant event auditing by his primary care team.

Introduction

We all enjoy a good discussion about a patient. We find people, and their healthcare, interesting; chatting about cases exploits that interest. Sometimes, a colleague will say something during such a case discussion that makes us raise our eyebrows. We want to know more, but feel we cannot probe without sounding challenging.

Yet, locked within these clinical case histories is the richest material: for expanding our knowledge and understanding; for our education and professional development; and for improving care for our patients. The unlocking of that rich seam is called 'significant event auditing'.

The technique simply offers a structure for case discussions, giving permission for colleagues to delve and enquire, and for the team to strive together to learn from each other's experience.

Two illustrative cases

The following two cases, in which details have been altered to protect confidentiality, are taken from routine primary care. The first illustrates the problems of a GP under stress.

Case number 1: a urinary infection

Mr Paul Mathews, aged 47, presented urgently at the front desk with frequency and pain on urinating. The receptionist 'fitted him in' with a doctor who was already running half an hour late. The doctor asked for a specimen and saw another patient while Mr Mathews passed urine. The doctor then examined the urine, finding clear evidence of a urinary infection. She prescribed amoxycillin and asked the patient to submit another urine specimen in two weeks' time.

Three days later a colleague was asked to visit Mr Mathews, who had a sustained florid allergic reaction to amoxycillin. Mr Mathews knew he was allergic to penicillin, but had not been asked specifically about that fact. He had not realised that amoxycillin was a penicillin. The allergy risk was not in Mr Mathew's computer record, nor written on the cover of the paper record. (A previous episode was recorded on a continuation card deep within the paper record.) This (second) partner arranged an x-ray of Mr Mathew's urinary tract. The test demonstrated a mass in the right kidney, which turned out to be a cancer.

Most GPs would recognise two lapses in good medical practice in the above. First, the possibility of penicillin allergy should be considered whenever a penicillin is to be prescribed. The doctor, under pressure, did not ask, but relied on the allergy alert in the computer's prescribing module. As it transpired, the computer record was incomplete because the computer entries had been taken from the front of the manual records – and Mr Mathew's allergy was not recorded on the record envelope.

When the primary care team discussed this case at its significant event meeting, the false reassurance from the computer's failure to alert the doctor, the dog that didn't bark in the night, was raised. The problem of relying on decision support when it fails to support you was highlighted. It was agreed to ensure that all patients prescribed penicillin were asked about allergies, regardless of the absence of a computer warning.

The second problem was the failure of the doctor to investigate a middle-aged man with a urinary tract infection. The doctor explained that she had intended to start investigations at a subsequent consultation, but no firm arrangement had been made for such an appointment. She agreed to review the literature, and to draft practice guidance on how to handle urinary infections in both men and women of all ages. That protocol was agreed at a later meeting and has been audited regularly since.

The practice discussion moved on to consider doctors' stress and, in particular, the fitting in of extra patients in a busy surgery. This topic came up recurrently over the next six months and culminated in a redesign of the appointments system. The doctor 'on-call' for emergencies on any given day would be given protected free appointments in each surgery, to cope with patients who could not wait until the end of surgery to be seen.

So, this one case: led to a clinical policy decision; a literature review and a new protocol; standard setting for clinical audit; and a change in the appointments system!

The second case concerns a complaint, where the practice could not defend the care that an elderly patient (at considerable risk) had received.

Case number 2: a complaint

The practice received a letter of complaint from Mrs Allsop's daughter, Beryl. Beryl had telephoned for a visit for her mother and was told a doctor would visit. Since nobody visited that day, she called again the next day and the GP registrar called. He listened carefully to Mrs Allsop's symptoms, examined her thoroughly, and explained that he felt there was 'nothing much the matter'. He arranged for a nurse to visit to take a blood test, which she did that afternoon.

Almost one week later, Beryl became very concerned about her mother and called the surgery on a Saturday afternoon. The duty doctor from the cooperative called and was concerned about Mrs Allsop's breathlessness and pallor. He arranged an emergency admission, where severe anaemia was diagnosed. After transfusion and stopping her arthritis tablets, Mrs Allsop returned home.

The primary care team discussed this case in some detail. First, the reception staff explained the circumstances around the failure to visit. A senior receptionist had taken the message but, being immediately distracted, had failed to write it down. After several subsequent meetings with the staff, it was agreed that one receptionist would take all telephone messages, other than requests for appointments, for the first three hours after morning surgery opening. No visit request has been missed since.

The doctors congratulated the GP registrar on his care during the home visit. His questioning and examination had been exemplary. He had arranged an appropriate investigation. Where care had fallen down was in responding to the faxed result, which had shown a very low haemoglobin. This result had been placed, with the notes, on the GP registrar's desk. He, however, had been absent for one day and, on his return, assumed that action had been taken, and that the result was merely there for information.

Clearly, something needed to be done to ensure this never recurred. A new policy was agreed whereby all faxed results would go to the duty doctor, who would liaise with the patient's doctor to ensure that appropriate action was taken. The duty doctor would also check all incoming pathology results for any highly abnormal results. It would be that doctor's responsibility to ensure that appropriate action was taken.

The practice manager wrote to Beryl setting out the content of the practice team's discussion and explaining the actions that resulted. Beryl visited the practice and discussed her mother's care with the practice manager and one of the doctors. She accepted the full apology of the practice and, in the light of the action that the practice had taken, did not pursue a formal complaint.

What do these cases tell us?

The primary care team discussed the two cases as 'significant events'. At monthly significant event audit meetings, the case notes of all patients with a major new diagnosis, or where care is a problem, are discussed. Such meetings offer the team insight into clinical and administrative failings.

Many primary care staff would prefer to sweep such cases under the carpet. Others fear that an open discussion of their care would result in ridicule and shame. Certainly such a discussion does require a cohesive team prepared to avoid finger wagging and the allocation of blame. The culture must be one in which a commitment to high-quality care is accompanied by a willingness to improve.

These two cases led to major changes in practice. Through such open discussion, team members learn how to avoid repeating mistakes and the team is able to minimise the risk of a formal complaint being lodged.

This is not an idealised vision of quality assurance. Primary care teams up and down the country already carry out significant event auditing. Later in this chapter personal experience of the process within one team is described. Before that, terms need to be defined and the background to significant event auditing examined.

Some definitions

Significant events are those that can be used to give an understanding of the care that an individual or team delivers. They may demonstrate good or less good care. Thus, a 63-year-old man being diagnosed as having rectal carcinoma is 'significant'. In reviewing the case notes it might become clear that best care was delivered. His family history was recorded and his higher risk noted. On presenting with rectal bleeding the doctor had done a rectal examination and referred him urgently. The hospital had responded quickly and his operation was performed within a month of presentation. He had been seen after discharge and potential family risks and screening had been discussed with his relatives.

More usually, however, at least some elements of care are found to be less than perfect. If this man had been treated with suppositories for his 'haemorrhoids' for several months before the diagnosis was made, the team could discuss the difficulties of diagnosis in rectal bleeding and how to avoid delay in future. While all significant events have the capacity to identify areas for improvement, most can also demonstrate good or appropriate care.

Some significant events are *adverse events*. These are events where something clearly has gone wrong, and the team needs to establish what happened, what was preventable and how to respond. Adverse events, therefore, might include, as in the two illustrative case studies, a patient complaint, an allergic reaction to a drug which was already known about, a visit request taken but the visit not done, a prescribing error, and so on.

A *critical incident* is a half-way house. It is an event that might indicate sub-standard care, but might also occur by chance. The presumption is, however, towards less good care. Any allergic reaction to a drug would be a critical incident, with the investigation aimed to establish whether it was avoidable. Other critical incidents might be an osteoporotic fracture, a stroke or a teenage pregnancy, all theoretically avoidable and all possible pointers to deficiencies in care.

Of the three options, it is preferable to use the term significant event auditing. It covers both adverse and critical events, is couched in more acceptable language, and its methodology encourages the identification and celebration of good care as well as exposing the bad. Conceptually it is in tune with the principles of adult learning, and psychologically it is less likely to provoke a defensive response.

Behind these terms lies the concept of *risk management*[1] (*see* Chapter 8). In every consultation there is a chance that the process of care might be sub-optimal. Risk management is the process by which that chance is reduced. Significant event auditing is a method for reducing clinical risk. Efficient administrative systems, a good complaints procedure, decision support, conventional auditing, error trapping (double-checking of prescriptions) and a positive culture with regard to quality are all valuable in risk management.

Inevitably, all of us could do better. We can, therefore, use significant event auditing to gather insight for personal development. Cases can feed into educational needs and personal and practice development plans. By studying the care delivered by other members of the team, we can identify ways in which patients may be put at risk, and we can personally, and as teams, work to minimise that possibility. If something has gone wrong, we can determine how to respond, often with an apology and action to ensure that it is unlikely to happen again. If the ultimate risk for health professionals is a formal complaint, significant event auditing reduces that risk. If the risk for patients is less than ideal care, this system helps to minimise that.

The background to significant event auditing

Significant event auditing is not new. Much of our core medical knowledge comes from descriptions of single cases or of a small series of cases. The links between clinical signs and pathology were established through postmortems. A well-conducted ward round can be seen as a 'prototype significant event audit meeting', with sharing of experience and knowledge and a striving for excellence.

While primary care opted to concentrate on clinical auditing of cohorts of patients, our hospital colleagues refined the perinatal mortality meeting into the confidential enquiry into maternity deaths.[2] There is now an expanding range of such enquiries, including those into peri-operative deaths, asthma deaths,[3] suicides[4] and deaths following accidents.[5] Increasingly, these enquiries involve examining care outside hospitals as well.

When the idea of auditing 'significant events' in primary care was first published[6,7] it appeared radical because it ran counter to the prevailing culture. It has become increasingly clear, however, that it was a concept that was mouldable to meet a range of needs. One of the uses most widely published has been the examination of case records following death.[8–10]

Basically, any systematic examination of individual case records, in an attempt to improve care for others, can fly under this banner. Some practitioners, for example, have reflected on cases where patients have made complaints.[11] There is a strong belief, admittedly based on anecdote rather than research, that openness in handling complaints, even to the extent of telling patients when they have experienced negligence, will ultimately protect the clinician.[12]

The technique has been used to explore: the interval between a patient first presenting with a symptom, which in retrospect was the first sign of cancer, and action being taken[13]; the processes underlying difficult prescribing decisions[14]; and the use of investigations.[15] In other countries it has been used to reflect on 'near misses' and adverse events, some of which are avoidable.[16,17]

One study used significant event auditing techniques to throw light on why significant event auditing may work.[18] One hundred clinicians, half of whom were GPs, were asked to discuss recent changes in their clinical practice. They reported an average of three reasons per change, neatly fitting the concept of triangulation. This suggests that we usually change our behaviour after reinforcement from three sources. A speaker at a lunchtime seminar says that all patients with a stroke need a scan to establish whether it is a bleed or a clot; a leader in a well-respected journal says the same thing; and, in discussion about a patient who has had a stroke, the district nurse says it is policy in the neighbouring practice to admit all strokes. Three similar messages delivered in different ways, and clinical behaviour changes.

So significant event auditing has a long tradition, but mainly in secondary care settings. It makes use of the rich learning material in clinical records; and it can be adapted to examine any aspect of care. It does, however, need a supportive team without a culture of blame. It needs a willingness to reflect and improve, as espoused in the concept of lifelong learning; and, if used effectively, it may reduce the risks of working in high-risk clinical professions.

Significant event auditing by one primary care team

One particular death in the treatment room in our practice triggered our team's interest in regular significant event auditing. Although three doctors attempted resuscitation, the patient died. In our subsequent discussions we felt that, given the size of the infarction, resuscitation was hopeless. But we recognised a whole range of issues that we had to address. These varied from skills in cardio-pulmonary resuscitation (CPR), through the maintenance of equipment, to the non-availability of a defibrillator.

One case, albeit a dramatic one, resulted in a wide range of changes. Over ten years ago, therefore, we started meeting every two months and, after a few meetings, monthly. We identify new cases (*see* Box 9.1) of myocardial infarction, stroke, unplanned pregnancy and cancer from the computer; acute admissions for asthma, diabetes and epilepsy are noted from hospital discharge sheets; complaints, prescribing errors, delayed diagnoses and administrative foul-ups are picked up by all of us. Any member of the

Box 9.1:   Potential significant events

- New cases of myocardial infarction.
- New cases of stroke.
- Unplanned pregnancies.
- New diagnoses of malignancy.
- Acute admissions for asthma, diabetes or epilepsy.
- Patients' complaints.
- Prescribing errors.
- Delayed diagnoses.
- Administrative 'foul-ups'.

primary care team can list any case for potential consideration, and we usually have between 10 and 15 to consider every month.

The meeting lasts one hour over lunch – sandwiches are used as an incentive, although being the most popular of our team meetings, an incentive is probably unnecessary. The doctors, practice and community nurses, and managers start by reviewing the decisions made at the last meeting. The team then discusses relevant patients and events, going around the room until everybody has had a chance to make a contribution.

Some discussions are very short. A 16-year-old girl has had a termination of pregnancy. She had been on the contraceptive pill and we have documented that she knew about post-coital contraception. The operation was arranged quickly and satisfactorily and she is now on the pill again. Opportunities for prevention were taken; care was good; the team is congratulated and the discussion moves on.

Some discussions are, however, lengthy. A 56-year-old has come home after a myocardial infarction. Did we know about his smoking, alcohol, body mass index, exercise and family history? Had we offered lifestyle advice? Does he come within the guidelines for screening for lipids? If so, was it done? Who attended the acute event and were they fully equipped? What has been done about rehabilitation?

There are four possible outcomes from these discussions, and often they occur together from the same case (*see* Box 9.2). First, and most importantly, significant event auditing can identify good practice. How often do we congratulate our colleagues on good care? A patient attended the nurse for a 'flu vaccination. The nurse noticed that the

Box 9.2:   Outcomes from significant event auditing

- Good practice identified and acknowledged.
- Further investigation carried out, e.g. literature review.
- Immediate change implemented.
- No lessons to be learned – normal primary care.

patient was pale and a little breathless. She took a full blood count that showed a chronic leukaemia. The team recognises and congratulates her on her initiative.

The second outcome is to investigate the situation further. This may take the form of getting advice from another doctor, performing a literature review, seeking out a guide-line, or talking to the patient and the family. Precipitate action in response to an event may be unwise; failing to reflect on what may have happened is equally unwise. This link between events and the educational needs of individuals and the whole team is, in our experience, very powerful.

Third, we may agree that immediate change is required. A doctor gave an injection on a home visit and only afterwards discovered that the drug was out-of-date. Fortunately the patient has come to no harm, but clearly this cannot happen again. It is decided to institute a system for regularly checking all drugs in doctors' bags. At the next meeting the team check that the new system is in place and working.

The last outcome from our discussions is to agree that there are no lessons to be learned. The case illustrates normal primary care, and there are no particular features to be discussed in depth. These are the most common cases but they cannot necessarily be identified in advance.

Our team is now very experienced in handling significant event audit meetings, but we have learned to abide by certain rules. Any primary care team setting out to under-take significant event audit would be well-advised to follow the guidelines (*see* Box 9.3), and the role of the chair (or external facilitator if used) is critical (*see* Box 9.4).

Box 9.3:   Guidelines for significant event audit meetings

- In general, cases chosen will have had a poor outcome or a 'near miss'.
- It is not an appropriate technique where legal action is anticipated or where individual incompetence is suspected.
- All the members of the relevant multidisciplinary group involved in the care should participate.
- The aim is to be supportive to team members – all feedback should be constructive not negative.
- It is not an attempt to search for the 'right way', but a means of exploring possible alternatives for the future.
- The chair (or external facilitator if used) should not have been actively involved in the case under discussion.
- A brief anonymised written summary of the case can be made available at the meeting providing key dates and relevant factual information.
- The case should be introduced by a brief presentation from the involved team member(s).
- The chair should compile a written summary of the general conclusions with any actions to be taken, for review at a future specified date.
- The chair's summary should be the only record of the meeting.
- Individual team members' actions in the care of the case and their contributions to its discussion at the meeting should not be discussed outside the meeting.

> **Box 9.4:   Role of the chair (or external facilitator if used)**
>
> - To explain the aims and process of the discussion.
> - To structure the discussion – that is, to keep to time, to encourage contributions from all participants, and to clarify and summarise frequently.
> - To maintain the basic ground rules of group discussion, for example, to allow uninterrupted discourse, to encourage participants to speak for themselves (using 'I' not 'we'), and to maintain confidentiality.
> - To clarify suggestions for improvement and identify who will be responsible for initiating change.
> - To recognise, acknowledge and enable appropriate expression of emotion within the group.
> - To remain 'external' to the group and to avoid giving unwarranted opinions or colluding with the group during discussions.
> - To compile a written summary of general conclusions with any actions to be taken, for review at a specified later date.
>
> Adapted from Robinson LA *et al.* (1995) *BMJ.* **311**: 315–18.

Conclusions

Significant event auditing encompasses a range of techniques for examining and learning from individual cases. It is a team activity and requires a mature and committed team. There is increasing evidence that, when used properly, it can be an effective catalyst for promoting quality of care and professional development. It can also help primary care teams to manage their risks, reducing the potential for things to go wrong in future. And it is clearly linked to evidence-based practice and the adoption of guidelines and best practice.

These characteristics make it an ideal feature of clinical governance. Significant event auditing can be the method at the centre of reflective practice, keeping up-to-date and responding to patients. But it is not enough on its own. Just as a calorie-controlled diet needs to be combined with exercise to achieve weight loss, so significant event auditing works best when it is part of a quality culture applied through a range of mechanisms. Significant event auditing cannot replace, for example, conventional cohort auditing, but it gives it added power.

The last note is, hopefully, redundant at this point in the chapter. Most doctors and nurses in primary care are motivated by an interest in people and a desire to improve health. Significant event auditing connects them with real people in a way that a table of results in a conventional audit cannot. That emotional content is why significant events are interesting, and why discussing them is effective. Change is an emotional process and significant event auditing uses emotional engagement to achieve improvements in patient care and make them stick.

Practical points

- Significant event auditing is a technique that provides a structured approach to case discussions.
- General lessons can be learned from individual cases.
- The term 'significant event' is preferable to 'critical' or 'adverse' event, and covers both.
- Significant event auditing is an effective means of reducing clinical risk, and promoting quality of care and professional development.
- It requires a mature and committed team with a supportive, reflective and no-blame culture.

References

1 Vincent C (1997) Risk, safety, and the dark side of quality. *BMJ.* **314**: 1775–6.

2 Hibbard B and Milner D (1994) Reports on confidential enquiries into maternal deaths: an audit of previous recommendations. *Health Trends.* **26**: 26–8.

3 Mohan G, Harrison B, Badminton R, Mildenhall S and Wareham N (1996) A confidential enquiry into deaths caused by asthma in an English health region: implications for general practice. *British Journal of General Practice.* **46**: 529–32.

4 Matthews K, Milne S and Ashcroft G (1994) Role of doctors in the prevention of suicide: the final consultation. *British Journal of General Practice.* **44**: 345–8.

5 Hussain L and Redmond A (1994) Are pre-hospital deaths from accidental injury preventable? *BMJ.* **308**: 1077–80.

6 Pringle M, Bradley C, Carmichael C, Wallis H and Moore A (1995) Significant event auditing. Occasional Paper 70. RCGP, London.

7 Pringle M and Bradley C (1994) Significant event auditing: a user's guide. *Audit Trends.* **2**: 20–3.

8 Robinson L, Stacy R, Specer J and Bhopal R (1995) Use of facilitated case discussions for significant event auditing. *BMJ.* **311**: 315–18.

9 Khunti K (1996) A method of creating a death register for general practice. *BMJ.* **312**: 952.

10 Holden J, O'Donnell S, Brindley J and Miles L (1998) Analysis of 1263 deaths in four general practices. *British Journal of General Practice.* **48**: 1409–12.

11 Pietroni R and de Uray-Ura S (1994) Informal complaints procedure in general practice: first year's experience. *BMJ.* **308**: 1546–8.

12   Ritchie J and Davies S (1995) Professional negligence: a duty of candid disclosure? *BMJ*. **310**: 888–9.

13   Holden J and Pringle M (1995) Delay pattern analysis of 446 patients in nine practices. *Audit Trends*. **3**: 96–8.

14   Bradley C and Riaz A (1998) Barriers to effective asthma care in inner city general practice. *European Journal of General Practice*. **4**: 65–8.

15   Robling M, Kinnersley P, Houston H, Hourihan M, Cohen D and Hale J (1998) An exploration of GPs' use of MRI: a critical incident study. *Family Practice*. **15**: 236–43.

16   Britt H, Miller G, Steven I *et al*. (1997) Collecting data on potentially harmful events: a method for monitoring incidents in general practice. *Family Practice*. **14**: 101–6.

17   Bhasale A (1998) The wrong diagnosis: identifying causes of potentially adverse events in general practice using incident monitoring. *Family Practice*. **15**: 308–18.

18   Allery L, Owen P and Robling M (1997) Why general practitioners and consultants change their clinical practice: a critical incident study. *BMJ*. **314**:870–4.

CHAPTER TEN

Lessons from complaints

Arthur Bullough and Ruth Etchells

When people cease to complain, they cease to think

Napoleon I

This chapter explores current complaints procedures which mainly affect general practitioners, and offers lessons that can be learnt from complainants both locally and in the wider NHS.

The context: current complaint structures and their history

Complaints procedures: necessary (resented) evil or ineffective good?

Few aspects of the NHS rouse stronger feelings in both clinicians and patients than the issue of appropriate complaints procedures. And all sides accept that mechanisms must exist for handling patient dissatisfaction efficiently and effectively. After all, the NHS should be accountable to the public. Yet, many GPs would also ruefully argue that the same need exists for handling their own complaints against patients.

- *A working definition of a complaint is 'any expression of dissatisfaction that needs a response'*

- *Information from complaints is free feedback about your service. This is the best form of market research you can get.*

From 'How to deal with complaints', Cabinet Office

Both public services and commercial organisations recognise that handling complaints *well* can bring immense benefits; and this is perhaps the first and most important lesson to learn from complaints. They make available important information about the current style of practice in a particular locality or practice, and used positively, a good complaints procedure can help individual doctors, the whole practice team or even a whole health authority not only avoid similar situations elsewhere but improve services generally. At the very least, it can save time and resources which would otherwise be spent on protracted disputes, and it *should* lead to improvement in practitioner/patient relationships across the board.

'Necessary evil?'

'Should' ... Ay, there's the rub. For it has to be faced that there remains (although far less sharply than with the pre-1996 process) a dichotomy between the GPs' perception of the complaints process and that of the public in general, and complainants in particular. Many GPs and primary care teams are hard pressed by a variety of administrative and legislative demands; needing to keep up with the fast-moving pace of developing medical research; pushed to meet the ever-increasing demands of patients; and wanting to effect preventive medicine but lacking the resources in time or staff to do so. To find themselves the target of a complaint is to feel themselves unjustly put on trial, however informal the process. So, to many, the government-imposed complaints procedure may indeed be 'necessary', but feel 'evil', in that, even if it does not go on to the now rare formal disciplinary hearing, it can be perceived as unfair, even threatening, and can cause much stress.

Case 1

A local health authority was told by Complainant Z that there had been no acknowledgement of the complaint, made in writing to the GP concerned, about the medical care offered to a spouse during what proved to be a terminal illness. Doctor A, when contacted about this, stated he had received no such letter. A second copy was sent, copied also to the health authority, from which it was clear the complaint lacked serious substance. When nothing had been heard from Dr A by either complainant or health authority, the latter contacted him in order to offer reassurance and help, only to hear with dismay that Dr A had felt so stressed on receiving the complaint that it had seemed to him to make his professional life unendurable, and he had that very day resigned from the practice.

'Ineffective good?'

Conversely, complainants feel that they are at a disadvantage when making a complaint. They often show themselves to hold an ambivalent attitude to their GP. Partly, this arises from a widespread sense of inequality with their doctor, who is often much better educated, more articulate and more socially confident than they. Their doctor is in some sense their 'judge' whenever they ask for clinical help. The relationship often starts to go wrong when the patient feels that the *manner* of the GP towards them is abrupt or dismissive or demeaning. At the same time it is clear from the tenor of many complaints we have processed that patient expectations of the medical profession have increased, and in many cases are unrealistic – sometimes wholly unreasonable.

The GP is (still) assumed by many to be properly available 24 hours a day, however minor the case. More deeply, there is an assumption, unexamined but clearly evident in many of the cases we have explored, that if only the GP were 'doing the job properly', the patient would not have suffered as he/she did, would have recovered more quickly, more fully, would not have died ... Add to this cocktail of social anxiety and clinical expectation the emotions of bereavement – grief and anger, and even unexplored guilt, which complainants sometimes bring to the process – and it will be obvious why on occasion the procedure seems to the complainants like a 'good' which doesn't deliver the goods. To them it is 'ineffective' because it could never in fact meet such a complex set of needs.

Against this background of strongly contrasted needs, hopes and fears, of the GP on the one hand and the complainant on the other, the government reassessed what a complaints process should attempt to achieve, and what it could not; how complaints might be better processed – more effectively, less stressfully and more quickly. Behind any attempt to set up a more effective complaints procedures there are contrasting principles, and we need to be aware of what these are in the present system.

New approach needed?

The present complaints procedure, which the government brought into effect in April 1996, after much taking of evidence, was based on two major principles, which differed sharply from what had gone before. First, and most fundamental, was the separation of complaints from disciplinary procedures. *A complaint sustained no longer implies breach of contract.* This clearly rejects the principle (tacitly held by some members of the general public and assumed by GPs) that a complaints procedure must in some sense be punitive in its intention. As long as this notion pervaded the process, it was inevitable that GPs would be thrown on the defensive, and find it difficult to engage whole-heartedly in co-operative discernment. Yet this is what effective complaints procedures really require.

Moreover, because of the quasi-judicial nature of the proceedings under the previous system, it was difficult for doctors to make any kind of personal apology for something that with hindsight could have been handled better. Often an apology was all that was actually required. It would have restored some kind of dignity in the doctor/patient relationship, and offered recognition that all had not been done, or said, well, causing the complainant (or the patient on whose behalf the complainant spoke) unnecessary distress.

Local resolution: 'owning' the process

The second major change was that complaints should always be dealt with informally, in the first instance, at practice level. The two governing principles here, new to the process, are subsidiarity and informality. The procedures are therefore much more immediate and accessible, inviting a combined effort from doctor and complainant, both of whom are invited to 'own' the process in an attempt to resolve the issue (*see* Box 10.1). This is cooperative discernment. Where this is not successful, other strategies are offered by the local health authority, still at an informal level. Only in the rarest cases should the matter go before a formal review panel.

Box 10.1:   The key objectives in the 'local resolution process'

- ease of access for patients and complainants
- a simplified procedure
- separation of complaints from disciplinary procedures
- making use of information from complaints to improve services
- fairness to staff and complainants alike
- more rapid, open process
- prime aim of resolving the problem and satisfying the concerns of the complainant

---

The present complaints procedures: the structure

A diagram of the current complaints procedure is given in Figure 10.1.

Since 1996 all practices have been required to have an in-house complaints procedure, the details of which are clearly publicised to their patients. They must:

- appoint a complaints manager, and an overseeing GP for clinical complaints
- draw up a complaints code of practice and ensure that staff follow it
- display a notice about the practice's complaints procedure and have leaflets available at reception.

Local resolution process, stage 1: complaints to practice

(a)   What about?

Anything! Premises, administration, delays, manner of reception, as well as clinical issues, are all legitimate material for complaint if they are felt to be less than

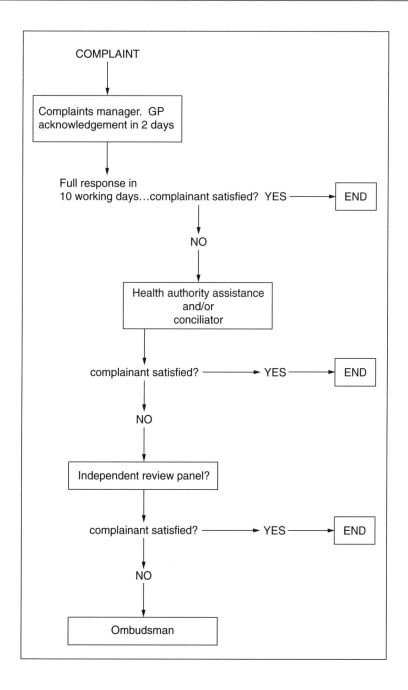

Figure 10.1   The complaints procedure.

satisfactory, since each is part of the total service offered. Sometimes a non-clinical matter is actually revealing of some quite serious difficulty within the practice itself.

Case 2

Complainant Y wrote to complain that the services being provided by Dr B had deteriorated significantly. The doctor was said to be spending less time with his patients, the practice premises were not being maintained to acceptable standards and practice staff were not being treated in an acceptable manner.

When this complaint was followed up it became clear that what could appear initially to be general apathy on the part of the doctor, went in fact far deeper. It was established that the reason for many of the problems was that Dr B was in dispute with a fellow GP who shared the premises. Many bills, for which the doctors had shared responsibilities, including gas and electricity, had not been settled.

What had begun as a complaint about a deterioration in service provision had revealed a serious professional situation between two GPs, which was undoubtedly having consequences for the services they offered.

There are regular occasions when receipt of a complaint by a health authority against a contractor can be indicative of other problems within a practice.

(b)   Who by?
      Patients, or former patients, of a practitioner who has arrangements with a health authority to provide family health services. Complaints may also be made on behalf of existing or former patients by anyone who has the patient's consent.

(c)   When?
      Normally within a period of six months of an incident occurring or within 12 months of it coming to light; discretionary extension is possible depending on the circumstances.

(d)   What happens?
      • Complaints are made orally, or in writing, to the practice and dealt with through whatever process the practice has set up.
      • An acknowledgement, or initial response, must normally be made by the practice within two working days.
      • An explanation, or more detailed response, must normally be provided within two weeks (i.e. 10 working days).
      • A careful record must be kept.
      • At the conclusion of all discussions the practice sends a letter to the complainant summarising all investigation, action and discussion which has followed the complaint.

(e) And if the complainant is not satisfied?
Sometimes the health authority complaints manager can, with the consent of both parties, act as 'honest broker' between GP and complainant in order to move the matter towards resolution. Indeed, if this is requested, such an intervention can take place at the earliest stage: particularly important if the complainant has no confidence in the practice's complaints procedures, or there is a strong personality clash. The resolution would still be taking place 'in-house', with the health authority merely acting as facilitator of the negotiations at practice level.

Should this fail, there is a further possibility.

Local resolution process, stage 2: conciliation process

Each health authority has available a number of trained conciliators, who can offer assistance whenever a practice or a complainant requests it. Their task is to facilitate agreement, and their work is therefore treated as wholly confidential. They must never be required to report to health authorities on the details of cases in which they are involved. Their role is most effective when used as early as possible in resolving complaints. Practices are wise to draw upon their expertise without delay if it seems that the complainant is resistant to, or dissatisfied with, the practice's first effort at resolution, even when the practice has been assisted by health authority personnel.

It is recognised that the normal *time target* of 10 working days to provide a full response to a complaint may need an *extension* if the services of a conciliator are deemed necessary.

If the matter still remains unresolved, even after the intervention of a conciliator, there is a further option for the complainant.

Stage 3: independent review panel

Complainants who remain dissatisfied after the local resolution process can ask the health authority convenor, either orally or in writing, for an independent review panel. The request has to be made within a given time limit.

It is the local convenor (appointed by the health authority from its non-executive members) who must decide whether an independent review panel is appropriate. The right to request one does not carry with it automatic consent. The convenor will always inform the GP of the request, and will ask for a copy of the final letter summarising action to date, together with the records kept by the practice of the whole process. The complainant must submit a letter setting out their remaining grievances, and why they are dissatisfied with the outcome of the local resolution process. The convenor must then, in consultation with an independent lay chairman appointed from a list held by the regional office of the NHS Executive and, where clinical issues are involved, a medical adviser, decide whether:

•   the GP or practice team can take any further action to satisfy the complainant

- the practice has already taken all practical action and establishing a panel would add no further value to the process.

In light of these the convenor will either agree to set up a panel, or not. Both complainant and doctor are advised of the decision and the reasons for it. Any panel will have the clinical advice of at least two doctors nominated by their professional bodies.

The chief objective of the panel is to resolve the grievance in a conciliatory manner, and it *may not make any suggestion in its report that anyone should be subject to disciplinary action*. To this conciliatory end it may determine for itself its method, choosing a style appropriate to the particular circumstances, and on no account allowing a confrontational situation to arise. For instance, the panel (never of more than three members) may meet with the complainant and the doctor separately; or it may decide on smaller meetings with only one member of the panel present to meet the two parties, although always with an assessor if a clinical matter is in debate.

The assessors will report in writing to the panel, which will normally attach such reports to its own final report, after checking a draft with the doctor and complainant to ensure factual accuracy.

The GP, complainant and anyone else interviewed by the panel next receive a copy of the final report. Where appropriate, the doctor may need to show parts of it to colleagues in the practice, whilst recognising its confidential nature. The health authority chairman and chief executive also receive the report, and the chief executive will write to the complainant about any action the health authority is taking as a result of the panel's work.

At the same time the complainant will be reminded that there remains a further stage, if they remain dissatisfied.

Stage 4: the ombudsman

Reference may only be made to the ombudsman when the NHS processes have been exhausted. The complainant may only move on to this stage, therefore, if they are either:

- refused an independent review panel

or

- dissatisfied with the work of the independent review panel set up at their request.

Lessons from complaints

Some statistics regarding complaints made in County Durham are given in Boxes 10.2 and 10.3.

Box 10.2:   Statistics 1997/98 – County Durham

Total number of written complaints against general medical practitioners	384
Resolved by practice	337 (88%)
Resolved following assistance from health authority and/or conciliator	40
Applications for independent review	7
Cases referred to ombudsman	0

Box 10.3:   Types of complaint 1997/98 – County Durham

General practitioners' manner and attitude	27%
Failure/incorrect diagnosis	26%
Refused home visit/delay in attending home visit	16%
Failure/refusal to refer or hospitalise	13%
Administrative concerns	14%
Receptionists/other staff	2%
Removal of patient from list	2%

What complainants want

There is a view that the majority of people who complain about their experiences of the NHS are seeking financial compensation. Studies have found that this is not so. Compensation is by no means the most popular motive. Rather complainants want:

* acknowledgement of the incident
* explanation in clear lay language
* an apology
* reassurance that preventive action will be taken to ensure no repetition.

More rarely people shift from wanting the GP to be accountable, to wanting consequent punishment. Compensation-seekers are similarly in this smaller group – indeed to some extent they coincide. In our experience fewer than 1% of complainants make it explicit that they are seeking financial compensation.

How to use a complaint positively

The most important lesson concerns attitude. What has emerged quite clearly from experience of complaints processes is that where doctors and other staff are receptive to complaints, and see them not as personal assaults but as information, indicators of a public perception and of possible improvement of services, really fruitful results can ensue.

For the individual, positive reactions would include the following list:

- Acknowledging the complaint quickly, always thanking complainants for bringing matters to the practice's attention.
- Sharing the matter with someone, colleague, local medical committee (LMC), practice manager, defence organisation and/or health authority complaints manager (who has a wealth of experience and can often help sort things out quickly).
- Working with the local community health council, to whom the complainant will often turn for advice and representation, remembering that resolving a complaint is a cooperative effort.
- While meeting the 10-day deadline for a full response after investigation, taking time before drafting it. (This gives opportunity for the first shock, and possibly anger, to be replaced by a calmer and more thoughtful approach; a tone more likely to engage with the complainant; and a thorough investigation and assembly of relevant documents.)
- Offering a meeting with the complainant, *but only if both complainant and practitioner* genuinely want it, and it has a clear purpose. (Disputing fact is rarely useful.)
- Writing a full response which is informative, truthful and in a language which will be understood. Some clinical terminology can have a radically different meaning for a lay person, and such misunderstandings can trigger or compound a complaint.
- Being prepared to say 'Sorry!'. If after investigation it seems that the standard of care was less than it should have been, an apology should be made. Our experience is that 'sorry' is the most useful tool in handling complaints.
  (NB: Many general practitioners fear they will admit liability if they apologise. It is for this reason, among others, that 'accountability' has been separated from 'liability' in the complaints process. The Medical Defence Union comments that a detailed explanation should always be given in response to complaints, and also an apology if it is recognised as appropriate. It does *not* constitute an admission of liability.)

For a practice team, positive reactions would include the following two points:

- Taking corporate responsibility for complaints, each team member giving support and encouragement to any member faced with a complaint. Our experience is that this is not always the case. The resolution of the complaint can then be more difficult, the doctor more distressed and the practice itself less effective.
- Taking any action found necessary to prevent repetition of the incident, outlining in their response their proposed remedies. It is unwise to guarantee the incident will not recur, but sensible to guarantee the situation will be kept under review.

Case 3

Complainant X's case concerned his wife, the diagnosis of whose cancer of the stomach and liver had been, in his view, unreasonably slow, pre-empting effective intervention, through what were perceived as inappropriate delays in referral on the part of the two GPs involved, Drs C and D. The history of the disease (as noted) began with visits to the surgery in January, February and March, with the patient complaining of 'wind' and dyspepsia and steady weight loss. Dr C's working diagnosis in March was of peptic ulcer or gallstones, although in view of the weight loss, she thought a malignancy possible. A blood test was arranged, not attended by the patient because of family commitments (her daughter had had a baby).

By April, new symptoms of cough (in a smoker) offered to Dr D prompted him to a tentative diagnosis of lung cancer. Under pressure, the patient attended a blood test (which proved normal) and a chest X-ray was urgently arranged, which also proved normal. This prompted Dr C to review her working diagnosis to one of upper gastrointestinal malignancy. After further blood and urine samples had been taken (which equally proved normal) she wrote to a consultant asking for an urgent appointment for the patient for assessment and further examination. Both Drs C and D were unaware there would be a four-week delay.

It was not, therefore, until the beginning of July that the patient had a hospital appointment; and not until 1 August was an endoscopy available. This, and a CT scan performed two days later, indicated an extensive gastric tumour, with further 'likely deposits' in the liver. No treatment was appropriate. The patient died in November.

Lessons for wider reference in the NHS

The health authority monitors all complaints (*see* Box 10.2) and takes note of any issues particular to the practice, which may have wider implications for primary care in general. (Case 3 above is a case in point.) Most health authorities arrange training sessions on complaints so that primary care team members can draw on what colleagues have learned from their experience of complaints. Practices are well advised to send a representative to these events.

Practices are also requested to undertake regular audits of patient complaints, and how these have been processed using in-house procedures. To widen the scope, complaints resolved immediately within the practice can be compared with those where conciliation or independent review is necessary. Practice guidelines can be developed and modified as a result, and outcomes fed back to the health authority on the one hand and the LMC on the other.

Many LMCs ask the health authority to keep them informed of issues raised through the complaints procedure.

And finally

Cooperative discernment of why things may have gone wrong, and how they can be improved, is no bad basis for learning from complaints.

Sources of information

Department of Health (1994) *Being Heard: the report of a review committee on NHS procedures.* HMSO, London.
NHSE (1996) *Practice-based Conflicts Procedure: guidance for general practices.* HMSO, London.

Practical points

- Handling complaints well brings benefits.
- Good complaints procedures provide free information about the practice.
- Protracted disputes cost time and money, and are very stressful to all concerned.
- Some practitioners take complaints too much to heart.
- Both practices and patients feel at a disadvantage within the complaints system.
- The complaints process separates complaints from disciplinary procedures.
- Often an apology by the practitioner is all that is needed.
- All practices must now appoint a complaints manager and an overseeing GP; have a complaints code of practice; and advertise the fact.
- Non-clinical complaints can reveal quite serious difficulties within a practice.
- Most complainants want reassurance that, if at all possible, what happened won't happen again.

CHAPTER ELEVEN

Tackling poor performance

George Taylor

We are what we repeatedly do; excellence, then, is not an act but a habit.

Aristotle

> The requirements of clinical governance are important not only for doctors, but for all those who work in primary care. This chapter initially focuses on doctors, but later deals with nurses and other members of the modern primary care team.

The individual doctor

Implications at a personal level

Although the term clinical governance is new, its components are not. Medical audit, learning from complaints and keeping up-to-date professionally, remain familiar to, and achievable by, each and every practitioner.

'The duties of a doctor'[1] are outlined by the GMC (*see* Box 11.1).

Allowing these principles to characterise an individual's work robs clinical governance of its dangers. No longer is it perceived as a threat. Rather, it is seen as a mechanism for ensuring the maintenance of personal and practice standards.

Indeed, all practitioners are aware of the need to keep up-to-date and to provide quality medical care. The government White Paper *A First Class Service: quality in the new NHS*[2] encourages all health service professionals to use the principles of clinical governance to underpin their own local arrangements for quality assurance.

Box 11.1: The duties of a doctor

- make the care of your patient your first concern
- treat every patient politely and considerately
- respect patients' dignity and privacy
- listen to patients and respect their views
- give patients information in a way they can understand
- respect the rights of patients to be fully involved in decisions about their care
- keep your professional knowledge and skills up-to-date
- recognise the limits of your professional competence
- be honest and trustworthy
- respect and protect confidential information
- make sure that your personal beliefs do not prejudice your patients' care
- act quickly to protect the patient from risk if you have good reason to believe that you or a colleague may not be fit to practise
- avoid abusing your position as a doctor
- work with colleagues in the ways that best serve patients' interests

---

The role of education

Informal mechanisms ensure that practitioners provide quality care on a daily basis. But what are these informal mechanisms? First, there are the questions which are thrown up in the course of everyday work. Such questions act as a trigger to refreshing knowledge and developing or refining skills. A simple example is the everyday question 'What is the dose of a certain drug?'. The action of looking up the answer in the British National Formulary, rather than guessing, is education.

Second, much audit work is done informally at a personal level. It is frequently not called audit, or even recognised as such. Wondering how many patients have had 'flu jabs begins an informal audit. Combine this with discussions about who should have 'flu jabs and then develop mechanisms to achieve such coverage, and it becomes both audit and education in action. Such activity involves collaboration with other team members and the development of practice standards.

Third, working with team colleagues to consider, and reflect upon, critical incidents, such as patient complaints or unexpected outcomes of care, leads to learning together. All such activities contribute to the success of clinical governance processes within the practice.

Individual GPs also have a responsibility to ensure that their continuing professional development is relevant to their 'needs' as well as their 'wants'. We all prefer to study areas that interest us rather than tackle topics that cause us problems. Developing a personal development plan, perhaps with the guidance of the local GP tutor, helps to avoid this tendency.

A number of enthusiasts will wish to undertake further methods of personal, professional development. For example, it is possible to assess the performance of oneself, and one's practice, against objective external measures of the quality of care being provided. There are a variety of ways of doing this. At a personal level, one can complete a higher degree at a local university or sit the examination to become a Member of the Royal College of General Practitioners. New mechanisms now exist for Membership or Fellowship of the Royal College of General Practitioners to be achieved by an assessment process.[3] This involves comparing personal and practice performance against nationally agreed standards in a developmental and constructive way. Most practitioners would feel that they gain far more from this type of activity than from the traditional educational method of sitting in a lecture theatre, being talked at by a local 'expert'.

Am I doing alright?

Yet some practitioners may worry that their performance at work is slipping. What might they do? Initially, they could seek advice from their local GP tutor, a senior practitioner whom they respect or the local health authority Director of Primary Care. General practice is slowly but surely embracing the concepts of both supervision and mentoring, approaches accepted as the norm in many stressful professions, such as social work and counselling.[4] By recognising areas of weakness, and in working to overcome them, rather than brushing them under the carpet, professionals gain in maturity and understanding.

Sadly, human nature dictates that many of us fail to recognise when we are underperforming, even when it is obvious to others that we are! Crude measures of performance, such as formal complaints from patients, will often fail to identify poor standards of care. Increasingly, professional colleagues have a responsibility to say if they feel that someone's performance is sub-standard, and that help should be sought.

The practice

Practices, like individual practitioners, have responsibilities both to themselves and to their patients. Achieving the highest possible standards is the goal for all. Yet, it is obviously disingenuous to expect practitioners working in a deprived inner-city area to be providing exactly the same type of care as those working in suburbia. The underlying concept, however, has to be achieving the highest possible realistic standards.

How can this be achieved?

The primary care team should review their work and reflect together on significant events in their practice, whether clinical situations or complaints from patients. In every situation, there is much to learn (*see* Chapter 8). Neither the doctor nor the patient is always right. Practices need to continue to develop their internal audit mechanisms. For audit is merely a tool to facilitate the development of quality care.[5] Primary care groups will no doubt use the existing expertise of medical audit advisory groups to develop district audits. Practices will increasingly need to compare their standards of clinical care with other local practices. There is an expectation that each practice will have a clinical governance lead, whose role will be to coordinate this type of activity.

Local accreditation schemes

National initiatives, such as the Kings Fund Organisational Audit[6] or the RCGP Quality Practice Award,[7] are external measures of quality which practices can use. Many will receive a 'pat on the back for good practice', whilst also being helped to highlight areas for future improvement.

Preventing underperformance

All practices have a responsibility to help team members who are underperforming. The traditional belief, that there are only two sorts of doctors, good doctors and very good doctors, is no longer tenable, and has not been for many years. Where a practice has anxieties about a member of its medical team, it should work together with that member to try to identify the causes of the problem and, if possible, help to rectify them. Some practices are developing internal appraisal systems, and this will undoubtedly help to facilitate personal development and the identification of areas for improvement.

Approaching the local GP tutors (with their associated educational network) for advice is, once again, a suitable route to follow to begin to solve problems before they become significant.

Medical practitioners in single-handed practice are in a unique professional situation. Whilst they can work with other team members to ensure good standards of practice, they will benefit from comparing their work with others. This can lead naturally to developing a system of supervision and appraisal, supported by local colleagues.

The clinical governance leads in each primary care group will have an important role in helping practices, particularly single-handed practices, to achieve the requirements of clinical governance. This will not be an easy task, and will take some years to develop.

Primary care groups

Primary care groups and, as they develop, primary care trusts, have a major responsibility for the development of quality of care. They will need to develop mechanisms which show a systematic approach to monitoring, and developing, clinical standards in practices within their geographical area. They will have to identify local and national priority issues, such as coronary heart disease, and develop quality standards in relation to them. They will need to have a supportive approach, enabling practices to compare their standard of healthcare with their neighbour's. The philosophy will be 'how can we help you improve' rather than 'we are going to beat you for not doing that'.

The difficult nettle that they will need to grasp is the identification of underperforming members within their local healthcare organisations. The first step must be to try and help underperforming practitioners identify that there are problems, and then provide supportive, educational guidance. There may well be situations, however, where a practitioner's performance leads to continuing anxiety and it becomes clear that the educational pathway may not be the correct one.

The ScHARR committee

All health authorities should, by now, have a local committee whose remit is to assess GPs whose performance gives concern.[8] Usually known as a 'ScHARR' committee (after the Sheffield University School of Health and Related Research, which developed the concept), this committee has a duty to review such cases of concern in a confidential manner. The usual composition of the group is:

- a senior health authority manager
- a senior local medical committee member
- a GP educationalist
- representatives of primary care groups or the local medical committee
- a lay health authority member.

Local factors may lead to some variation in this composition.

The ScHARR committee can consider information relating to any practitioner whose performance is causing concern. At one extreme, the committee may decide that there is no significant case to answer. They may then take no further action in the matter. At the other extreme, the committee may decide that the doctor in question has a significant and persisting problem with clinical performance. This would lead to a direct referral to the GMC by the ScHARR committee.

Where anxieties exist within the committee about a doctor's performance, but the extent of poor performance is unclear, then a local assessment is needed. This would usually be carried out by senior medical practitioners. Such an assessment seeks to identify significant needs. If these can be met through education, the doctor would usually be referred to the GP tutor or the local Director of Postgraduate General Practice Education. If a major problem is identified, the doctor would need to be referred directly to the GMC. Where the local assessment team feels unable to quantify the extent of

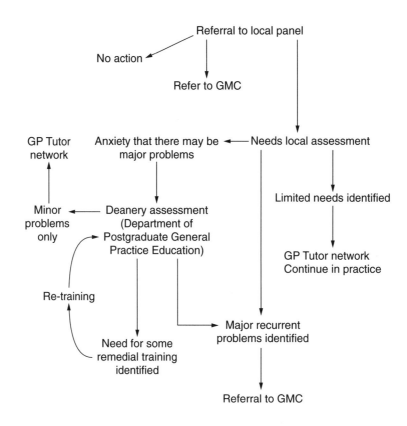

Figure 11.1   Pathways: the ScHARR committee.

underperformance, an educational assessment by the department of the Director of Post-graduate General Practice Education can provide the ScHARR committee with an educational prescription, if this is appropriate. This assessment may, once again, lead to direct referral to the GMC. The director may be able to direct doctors with problems to a suitable source of remedial training. If the problems identified are relatively minor, they will usually be dealt with within the local educational network. Figure 11.1 shows the pathways diagrammatically.

The General Medical Council performance procedures

No doctor ever wishes to be referred to the GMC. All doctors are, however, charged with ensuring the quality of medical care. 'Patients must be able to trust doctors with their lives and well being. To justify that trust we, as a profession, have a duty to maintain a good standard of practice and care and to show respect for human life'.[9] The GMC mechanisms for underperforming doctors are outlined in Figure 11.2.

As can be seen, this is a complex procedure that is also time-consuming. If the screening procedure suggests that there may be a case to answer, the doctor involved will be asked to complete a portfolio. This relates to medical experience, basic and continuing medical education, and day-to-day clinical practice. Following this, an assessment team

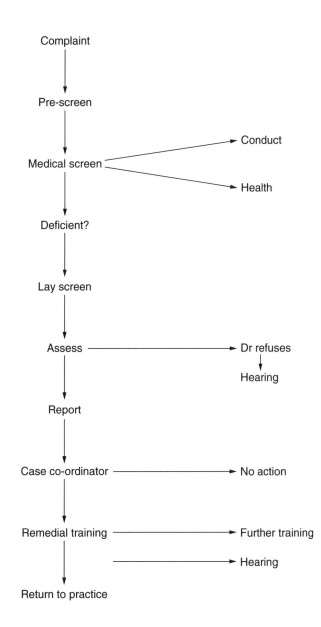

Figure 11.2   The GMC performance procedures (based on GMC document).

of experienced practitioners and trained lay assessors arrange a visit. They review all facets of care. This includes the structure of the surgery building, the doctor's consultation skills, relationships with patients and with other professionals, clinical management skills and the use of drugs. The visiting team's report goes to a case coordinator, who may identify suitable remedial action at this point. If the doctor agrees to such remedial action, then there will be no need for an appearance before the Committee on Professional Performance. If, however, serious underperformance is identified, an appearance in front of the committee will be required.

The remedial action identified by the case coordinator will be transmitted to the local Director of Postgraduate General Practice Education, who will direct the doctor to suitable sources of available retraining. The cost of funding this retraining rests with the involved doctor. It is likely that, in some cases, health authorities will contribute to this.

Following this period of remedial training, reassessment will take place and, if found to be satisfactory, the doctor will be able to return to practice. A further period of retraining may, however, be recommended. If no improvement has occurred, the doctor will appear in front of the performance committee of the GMC, and may lose his or her registration or be suspended.

The NHS Tribunal

In some extreme situations, a health authority or primary care group may be concerned that a doctor is continuing to practise in a dangerous fashion in relation to the health of patients. The suspension of a self-employed practitioner is both very difficult and a last resort. Hence, the first approach must be to advise such a doctor of the urgency of refraining from medical work voluntarily. The doctor does not, however, have to take this advice. In this situation, the NHS Tribunal should be considered. This body can authorise interim suspension of a practitioner when it is felt that patient care is at serious risk of being compromised.

Whilst this may seem an effective mechanism, in practice it is rarely used. It is not easy to obtain an order to suspend a practitioner and the legal mechanisms to be followed are very time-consuming. These matters are under consideration and a more effective process is likely to be found in the future.

Salaried doctors

It should be noted that one recent development in general practice is the increasing number of doctors who are salaried employees either of practices or of health authorities. They are often found in 'Career Start'-type posts.[10] As employees, these doctors have contracts which allow them to be suspended by their employer to enable investigation to take place. Suspension does not mean guilt. It merely means that investigation is being undertaken.

Increasingly, primary care groups and the primary care team may employ salaried doctors. It is essential that proper mechanisms are in place to monitor the performance of such doctors, and that both disciplinary and grievance procedures are clear and equitable.

Nurses

At present, nurses, be they district nurses, practice nurses, health visitors or midwives, are either trust or practice employees. As employees, they should have clear guidance from their employer about the mechanisms to be followed in the event of a complaint being made against them, or concerns expressed about their performance. Doctors and primary care groups should know the local procedures. In most situations, suspension would be the norm, where an incident is felt to be significant, to allow investigation to take place.

All individual nurses, whatever their nursing role, have exactly the same professional responsibilities as doctors to ensure that high standards of care are provided. Nurses working in a team also have responsibilities to each other. They should identify under-performance and help underperforming colleagues correct problems before they become significant. The implications of clinical governance apply equally to all members of the primary care team. Procedures similar to those in place for doctors will need to be in place to monitor standards of working and to provide formative feedback to enable development for all. Mechanisms for coping with significant underperformance, that require either suspension and/or referral to the UKCC, are also needed.

UKCC

At present, the United Kingdom Central Council for Nursing, Midwifery and Health Visiting (UKCC) is the regulatory body for the nursing profession. This body has procedures for monitoring health matters and discipline issues, but does not have a specific pathway for nurse performance. The Code of Professional Conduct, however, requires that each nurse, midwife or health visitor acts at all times: 'To report to an appropriate person or authority where it appears that the health or safety of a colleague is at risk, as such circumstances may compromise standards of practice and care'.[11] Nurses are also asked to 'assist professional colleagues in the context of your own knowledge experience and sphere of responsibility to develop their professional competence'. At the time of writing, the regulation of nurses, midwives and health visitors has been subject to a review. This review has recommended the establishment of a unified regulatory body for the UK which will be smaller in size than the UKCC.

As the current regulatory body for nursing, the UKCC must respond to complaints from employers, patients, colleagues or carers. Following a complaint, a case officer investigates, gathering evidence and statements over several months. A preliminary proceedings committee then decides whether there is a case to answer. This body includes lay representatives. This may lead to a referral on health grounds, a formal hearing or a warning. On rare occasions, interim suspension is invoked pending investigation if public safety or the practitioner's interests seem best served by this.

If the professional conduct committee finds against the nurse, removal from the register can follow. Situations of less major concern may lead to a caution for the nurse. In some cases, the case is closed, with no further action being taken.

In the interests of equity it would seem likely that primary care groups will develop mechanisms similar to those for doctors to identify poor nursing practice at an early stage.

Other professions related to medicine working within primary care

An increasingly large team nowadays contributes to the provision of primary care. For example, there are chiropodists, speech therapists, social workers and counsellors, to name but a few. Limitations in the size of this chapter preclude a full discussion of the disciplinary and performance mechanisms of these differing professional groups, but common themes still apply. The responsibility of any professional is to ensure that clinical practice is up-to-date and competent. Professionals working together have a common responsibility to ensure that all team members perform to a satisfactory level and to report significant underperformance to protect patients from inadequate care. As employees, these health professionals should have clearly laid out disciplinary mechanisms to be followed in cases of complaint. They also have national registering bodies with mechanisms for dealing with poor performance.

Conclusion

Most health professionals want to do a good job. They have a responsibility, both to themselves and to patients, to ensure that underperformance in colleagues is identified at a very early stage. If appropriate action is then taken, most problems can be dealt with in a caring and confidential manner. Practitioners who are felt to be underperforming significantly must be reported either to the local ScHARR committee or their employer as appropriate, or, if the situation is serious, to the GMC or relevant regulatory body.

Practical points

- It is the duty of all professionals to ensure that their clinical practice is up-to-date and competent.
- Professionals working in teams have a common responsibility to ensure that all team members perform satisfactorily.
- It is no longer acceptable to ignore poor performance in oneself or in others.
- Doctors are guided by the GMC's *Duties of a Doctor*.
- Each profession has its own regulatory authority.
- Both formal and informal education play their part in supporting good practice.
- Single-handed practice is a unique professional situation.
- Local ScHARR committees consider underperforming doctors.
- The GMC performance procedures and the NHS Tribunal should, ideally, be options of the last resort.
- Employers, be they practices or NHS trusts, must have clear procedures for tackling poor performance among employees.

References

1   General Medical Council (1995) *Duties of a Doctor*. GMC, London.

2   Department of Health (1998) *A First Class Service: quality in the new NHS*. Health Service Circular: HSC(98)113, Department of Health, London.

3   Royal College of General Practitioners (1995) *Occasional paper 50. Fellowship by assessment*. RCGP, London.

4   Rutt G and Batchelor H (1998) The doctor, the patient and the supervisor. *Education for General Practice*. **9**: 508–12.

5   Irvine D and Irvine S (1998) *Making Sense of Audit*. Radcliffe Medical Press, Oxford.

6   The Kings Fund (1994) *Kings Fund Organisation Audit*. King's Fund, London.

7   Royal College of General Practitioners (1997) *The Quality Practice Award*. RCGP, London.

8   Rotherham G, Martin D, Joesbury H *et al.* (1997) *Measures to Assess GPs Whose Performance Gives Cause for Concern*. University of Sheffield, Sheffield.

9   General Medical Council (1997) *The Performance Procedures: a guide to the new arrangements*. GMC, London.

10 Harrison J and van Zwanenberg T (eds) (1998) *GP Tomorrow*. Radcliffe Medical Press, Oxford.

11 United Kingdom Council for Nursing, Midwifery and Health Visiting (1992) *Code of Professional Conduct*. UKCC, London.

CHAPTER TWELVE

Continuing professional development

Janet Grant

This chapter describes how continuing professional development (CPD) is central to clinical governance, and needs to be managed. Effective CPD involves assessing educational needs, learning in a variety of different ways, and implementing and reinforcing that learning.

With the advent of clinical governance in primary care, continuing professional development (CPD) has moved centre-stage. As an important part of the risk management and quality assurance responsibilities of primary care groups, practices and individual clinicians, the way in which CPD is managed in primary care is a subject of interest to users, providers and managers of primary healthcare services.

The new framework for CPD has been laid out clearly in *A First Class Service*[1] and in the Chief Medical Officer's review of CPD in general practice.[2] The framework is consistent with both research on the effectiveness of CPD and with professional needs and approaches to continuing education.[3] It is generic and can, and should, be used to plan managed CPD for all members of the primary care team. The challenge set by the framework is not to develop new ways of learning in primary care, but rather to put into place a management process that will support the CPD that is undertaken and make it evident and relevant.

What is managed CPD?

CPD vs CME

Until recently, the learning that doctors undertook once they had completed their training was called continuing medical education (CME). However, three main factors have militated against the use of this term:

- the content areas which doctors now study
- the learning which clinicians share with other members of the healthcare team
- the need to make continuing education effective in developing and assuring standards of practice.

Although doctors will always continue to learn more about clinical medicine throughout their working lives, and to refine and develop their skills in that area, clinicians increasingly need to address areas which are not clinical at all. These might include information technology, management, audit and educational skills. These are professional rather than purely medical matters.

Doctors increasingly share areas of their continuing professional development with other members of the healthcare team. National interest groups and societies, for example in asthma or diabetes, have a multiprofessional membership. In practices, questions of management and some aspects of practice policy will be shared by the team as a whole or by certain members of the team. As far as government guidelines are concerned, the framework for CPD that is offered is one that can be applied to all members of the primary care team and to practices as a whole. It is therefore a framework that is for CPD, not for the continuing education of only one discipline. Systems of continuing education which simply ask for proof or an account of education undertaken, do nothing to ensure that the education is either derived from, or feeds back into, practice. This means that neither the individual nor the health service can be confident that educational time has been well spent. If education is to be linked to CPD, then it must be approached, planned and managed more effectively. The emphasis will shift from isolated education to education as part of CPD.

CPD is accordingly defined in *A First Class Service* as:

... a process of lifelong learning for all individuals and teams which meets the needs of patients and delivers the health outcomes and healthcare priorities of the NHS and which enables professionals to expand and fulfil their potential.

Managed CPD

Despite systems that have not required it, many doctors have assessed their own learning needs, have undertaken learning relevant to those needs, and have brought that learning back to the practice so that it influences quality of patient care or organisation within the practice. It cannot, however, be said that this has been the norm everywhere.

With clinical governance comes the need to ensure that all aspects of a clinician's work, and the work of the team, contribute towards a service of increasing quality, as the definition of clinical governance implies.[1]

The term 'accountable' in the definition makes it clear that if CPD is a significant part of clinical governance, then it is also a part that must be managed properly and openly, just as all other aspects of healthcare provision and organisation will be accountable and managed. In relation to that management, it is asserted that CPD programmes are best managed locally to meet both local service needs and those of the individual professionals.[1]

Therefore:

Health professionals, professional bodies and local employers need to discuss a locally-based approach to CPD, centred on the service development needs of the local community and the learning needs of the individual.

Managed CPD and clinical governance

A First Class Service states that clinical governance provides the framework for a more coherent approach to local CPD which will, in turn, support improvements in service quality.[1]

Its recommendations are quite explicit about where CPD fits into the clinical governance and quality framework. The importance of CPD and its role in quality assurance is reinforced by a recommendation that primary care groups should nominate a senior professional to take the lead on clinical standards and professional development, as part of the group's overall responsibility to demonstrate that quality of care is important.

The following specific points are made about CPD in relation to clinical governance:

- it must play a key part in improving quality
- individual health professionals and NHS employers should value CPD
- CPD programmes should meet the learning needs of individual health professionals as well as the wider development needs of the service
- professional bodies should support effective CPD and promote lifelong learning
- much good CPD is already in practice throughout the NHS
- CPD is essential to the development and support of clinical governance
- CPD programmes are best managed locally to meet the needs of individuals and the service. This might include innovative approaches to work-based learning
- the CPD cycle is made up of the five stages (*see* Box 12.1)
- employers must recognise the value of appropriately managed CPD programmes in attracting, motivating and retaining high-calibre staff
- personal development plans (PDPs) should be developed by individuals in discussion with colleagues locally, perhaps in the context of performance appraisal

---

Box 12.1:   **Five stages in the CPD cycle**

1   Assessment of individual and organisational needs.
2   Making personal development plans (PDPs).
3   Implementation.
4   Reinforcement and dissemination.
5   Review of the effectiveness of the CPD intervention.

- PDPs should take into account different preferred ways of learning and should take full advantage of opportunities to learn on the job
- individual PDPs should be complemented by organisational development plans
- the majority of health professionals should have PDPs in place by April 2000.

What does managed CPD involve?

From this, and from what is known about the effectiveness of CPD, we can say what managed CPD should mean in practice:

- each member of the primary care team should prepare a PDP
- the plan should record:
  - the need for the CPD to be undertaken
  - what the CPD will be
  - how that CPD will be reinforced and disseminated locally to show its effectiveness
- the PDP should take into account the needs of the individual and of the service
- the PDP should be prepared jointly by the individual and an appropriate colleague
- the PDP should form part of the Practice Professional Development Plan (PPDP) and so should be open to scrutiny and monitoring.

What makes CPD effective?

Before describing in more detail the nature of managed CPD in primary care, it is important to appreciate that there is an evidential basis for it.

The literature review[3] undertaken for the Chief Medical Officer in preparation for the *Review of Continuing Professional Development in General Practice*, came to the following conclusions:

- the key to effectiveness of CPD is not to be found in the learning methods adopted
- there is not a best learning method and no best approach to learning for CPD

- instead, the key to effectiveness is to make sure that the process of CPD is managed effectively and has the following components:
  - *a stated reason* for the CPD to be undertaken. This might be specific, e.g. a need to develop a new skill, or it might be a general professional reason, e.g. a wish to undertake general professional updating with colleagues at a conference. It might also arise from the needs of the service, e.g. to develop the skill to offer new areas of care to patients
  - *an identified method of learning* which might be formal or informal
  - *some follow-up* after the CPD for reinforcement and dissemination of the learning that can also demonstrate its benefits. This might be actions such as reporting back to colleagues, developing new services, demonstrating new skills or simply feeling more confident.

These conclusions match those of Davis *et al.*[4] in their review of randomised controlled trials of CPD interventions. Davis *et al.* elaborated on other reasons for success. In general, change was more likely where:

- a needs assessment had been conducted
- the education was linked to practice
- the educational activity was undertaken through personal incentive rather than other influence
- there were reinforcing features after the educational event itself.

This is not to imply that all education should be based on identified specific needs. General professional continuing education, such as the large conference that covers many topics, is an important part of CPD. If all education were specific and based on rigid needs assessment, the profession would be narrow in its perspective and its development.

Implications

The implications of the review are these:

- that a managed process for CPD must be developed at the practice level
- the *process of CPD* should be monitored and rewarded rather than the hours taken up by it
- the managed process must display the characteristics of effectiveness, being:
  - a stated reason for undertaking the intended CPD, i.e. a statement of learning needs and interests
  - an identified learning method, formal or informal
  - a plan for reinforcing and disseminating the learning and showing its effectiveness
  - a plan for review of the individual's PDP.

These implications are at the heart of the managed CPD which clinical governance requires.

Managed CPD in primary care

The principles of managed CPD apply to both primary and secondary care settings. In both cases, managed CPD must encompass the needs and interests of both the individual and the service. In hospitals, this can be done by integrating individual PDPs for CPD with the unit business plan. The equivalent of the unit business plan in primary care is sometimes called the Practice Strategic Plan. In primary care, however, where the educational needs of the whole team have been emphasised, a further planning stage is required to cover that whole team. This stage is summarised in the Practice Professional Development Plan (PPDP), as recommended in the Chief Medical Officer's report.[2] The levels of planning for CPD that are therefore recommended for primary care can be represented diagramatically (Figure 12.1).

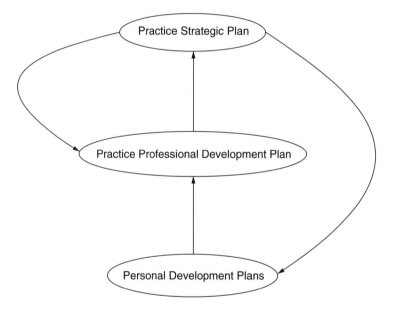

Figure 12.1   CPD planning in primary care.

The Practice Professional Development Plan (PPDP)

The PPDP addresses the learning needs of the whole practice and everyone in it. It is, in essence, the educational plan for the practice based on service development plans, local and national objectives and identified educational needs.

The PPDP is therefore practice based and should include an indication not only of what learning is required and planned for the practice, but also how its effect would be shown. In this way, the PPDP is partially based on the Practice Strategic Plan (or business plan) and feeds into that plan (*see* Box 12.2).

> **Box 12.2:** **Factors to be taken into account in PPDPs**
>
> - service developments
> - clinical audit results
> - local and individual needs
> - local and national priorities
> - user and carer involvement

The PPDP will allow practices to identify where both multiprofessional and uni-professional learning is required.

Personal development plans (PDPs)

Primary care has, in common with all branches of the health service, that the majority of staff should have a PDP by April 2000. The PDP must be a comprehensive document that records the outcome of appraisal, discussion of educational needs with a colleague or other forms of educational needs assessment. It has to be sufficiently detailed to be a clear part of the PPDP and to be monitored for professional or employment reasons. It is the main professional record of the individual's activities in keeping up-to-date and ensuring the standard and quality of the service provided. The PDP is an instrumental part of clinical governance and professional maintenance of standards, and is likely to be a key part of doctors' revalidation procedures.

A PDP should contain sections that record:

- what the planned CPD activity is
- its intended date of completion
- how the educational need was identified
- the reinforcement and dissemination activities planned after the CPD itself is completed
- dates of completion of the plans.

Fulfilment of the PDP can then be monitored.

An example of a PDP form is given in Figure 12.2.

The stages of managed CPD: identifying educational needs, learning and follow-up

There are three stages of managed CPD that the individual doctor will follow: needs identification, learning and follow-up (i.e. reinforcement, dissemination and showing effectiveness).

PERSONAL DEVELOPMENT PLAN			
DOCTOR:	PRACTICE:		
GMC NUMBER:	DATE:		
PLAN FOR PERIOD:	To		
PROPOSALS DISCUSSED WITH:	DATE OF DISCUSSION:		
Description and intended date		**Date completed**	**Signed by colleague [Date]**
1. Proposed CPD activity	Intended date:		Date:
How need was identified:			Date:
How CPD will be reinforced, and disseminated, showing effectiveness			Date:
2. Proposed CPD activity	Intended date:		Date:
How need was identified:			Date:
How CPD will be reinforced, and disseminated, showing effectiveness			Date:

A copy of this form should be lodged in the Practice Strategic Plan and be retained for future use in relation to monitoring.

Figure 12.2   Personal development plan.

The review of the effectiveness of CPD shows that these three stages are already being undertaken by many practitioners in many ways, and that these three stages together will ensure that CPD is effective for individuals and for primary care teams. Preparation of the PDP will enable practitioners to demonstrate this fact and to consider new methods of effecting these stages.

A research and development project has identified and described the various ways in which doctors are already undertaking these three stages of managed CPD. The following examples are taken from the report of that project.[5]

Methods of needs assessment

Forty-eight methods of needs assessment have been identified, as shown in Table 12.1.

Table 12.1 Methods of needs assessment used in medicine

The clinician's own experiences in direct patient care

- blind spots
- clinically generated unknowns
- competence standards
- diaries
- difficulties arising in practice
- innovations in practice
- knowledgeable patients
- mistakes
- other disciplines
- patients' complaints and feedback
- post mortems and the clinicopathological conference
- patient unmet needs (PUNs) and doctor educational needs (DENs)
- reflection on practical experience

Interactions within the clinical team and department

- clinical meetings: departmental and grand rounds
- department business plan
- department educational meetings
- external recruitment
- junior staff
- management roles
- mentoring

Non-clinical activities

- academic activities
- conferences
- international visits
- journal articles
- medico-legal cases

Table 12.1   cont

* press and media
* professional conversations
* research
* teaching.
* patient satisfaction surveys
* risk assessment

Formal approaches to quality management and risk assessment

* audit
* morbidity patterns
* patient adverse events

Specific activities directed at needs assessment

* critical incident analysis
* gap analysis
* objective tests of knowledge and skill
* observation
* revalidation systems
* self-assessment
* video assessment of performance

Peer review

* external
* informal: of the individual doctor
* internal
* multidisciplinary
* physician assessment

The following unusual methods might require some description.

PUNs and DENs

This method has been developed and used in general practice:

* PUNs = patient unmet needs
* DENs = doctor educational needs.

Richard Eve from Taunton, who developed the approach, recommends that a clinician collects PUNs during a set number of surgeries (outpatients, ward rounds, lists) simply by asking after each patient or session: 'Was I equipped to meet the patient's needs? Could I have done better?' Any clinician who thinks for a moment will be able to list many ways in which his or her practice has changed over the years. New drugs, new technology and equipment, new methods, procedures and techniques are always being introduced. Along with these comes the need to learn to use them properly and well. Acquiring the training or education to do so should be a high priority and properly planned. A note should be made of the answer to these questions: these will be the PUNs. In this way, an area or areas will be identified that might benefit from further learning or development: these will be the DENs. Eve points out that some PUNs will not be met by education but by changes elsewhere, such as in organisation or administration. For CPD, it is necessary to identify those PUNs which truly indicate a DEN and then act on them.

Professional conversations

Clinicians live in a rich daily professional learning environment that is dominated by discussion of patients and of practice. Clinicians in all disciplines discuss their own patients with other clinicians whose views are sought. They discuss shared patients and they discuss others' patients and experiences. These informal professional conversations are as much a part of learning and of identifying learning needs as any other type of more formal approach to needs assessment. Such professional conversations contain feedback on performance in relation to specific patients when the management or outcome of treatment is discussed. They also contain new learning and open up new areas for learning, which are often followed up quite deliberately. Where this is so, a learning need has been identified in a relevant and professional manner.

Gap analysis

Gap analysis is based on the idea that 'a learning need is the gap between what you are now and what you want to be in regard to a particular set of competencies'.[6]

Gap analysis is undertaken by:

- defining the knowledge, skills, attitudes and competencies which are required to perform the relevant role excellently
- defining where you are in relation to each aspect defined. This can be done either by you or with the help of others.

Physician assessment

This is a particular variant of peer review which came from the American Board of Internal Medicine[7] and was further developed by the Royal Australasian College of Physicians.[8] To undertake such an assessment, the doctor nominates a number of colleagues, say 15, to be assessors. Each is sent a standard rating form by the organising body (which could be the department, the trust or Royal College) and asked to rate the doctor on various clinical skills, humanistic and other qualities. The ratings are fed back to the doctor who takes educational action accordingly. The system shows encouraging levels of validity, reliability and acceptability and has the advantage of credibility to the doctor who has nominated the assessors. This is a form of 360° appraisal.

Methods of learning

Research on the effectiveness of CPD shows that the method of learning adopted is not the crucial variable for effectiveness. Clinicians learn in a rich variety of ways, many of which are integrated into their daily professional activities. Learning in healthcare is often not a separate event from practice itself. Practitioners live in a rich learning environment where contact with other healthcare professionals, with patients and with other information sources is built into normal working. These are powerful sources of education and development for the individual and the team. *The Good CPD Guide* describes over 40 such learning methods classified under the following headings:

- Academic activities
- Meetings
- Learning from colleagues
- Learning from practice
- Technology-based learning and media
- Management and quality-assurance processes
- Specially arranged educational events.

The many methods identified under these headings are not described further here. It is not the learning method that determines the effectiveness of the learning, but the stages of needs identification and reinforcement that go before and after it. Nonetheless, it is important that every clinician is able to identify the various ways of learning. They can then record them in their PDPs. In addition the learning which occurs in such ways can be undertaken perhaps more deliberately, consciously, critically and so more effectively.

Following up CPD: reinforcement, dissemination and showing effectiveness

Following up CPD has three main purposes. First, it reinforces the learning in the practice context. Second, it allows for dissemination of the learning to others in the practice, and third, it allows the overall effectiveness of the CPD to be judged.

These three purposes are different in their intent. Reinforcement will ensure that the primary learning is strengthened by its rehearsal or revisiting in some way. Dissemination allows the learning to be shared with others, discussed and analysed. Both reinforcement and dissemination might involve application of the learning to change or to develop practice. Demonstration of the overall effectiveness of the learning will often be a consequence or antecedent of the reinforcement and dissemination activities, but it might also be a special event.

Although the effectiveness of CPD can be demonstrated in many ways, hardly any of these will be able to produce a measurable outcome, or causal relationship between the education and the effect studied. This is for a number of reasons:

- On some occasions, the CPD will simply show that the clinician's practice is acceptable and does not require changing. The only 'measurable' outcome therefore might be increased confidence on the part of the clinician.
- Many important outcomes of education are unpredictable and, if they are predictable, are often unmeasurable, e.g. 'better team spirit'.
- Education is often not an isolated event but occurs in parallel with other educational influences. So isolating the effects of that event is difficult.
- Where education is a discrete event, there are often many interfering variables between event and patient outcome that might either militate against or facilitate the outcome observed. Attribution of that outcome to the education will therefore be impossible. The problem of measuring outcomes is discussed further in Grant and Stanton.[3]

Despite these difficulties, it should be remembered that the clinicians' professional judgement of unmeasurable qualities can be as valuable and valid as quantitative data that can measure only the measurable and thereby often miss the important.

The Good CPD Guide discusses 41 ways of following up learning, as shown in Table 12.2. It is crucial that this stage of the managed CPD process is not omitted.

Table 12.2   Methods of following up CPD

1 Accreditation/certification of the individual	22 Networking
2 Accreditation of services	23 New services
3 Appraisal	24 Obsolete and inappropriate practice
4 Assessment of learning	25 Peer review of the doctor's CPD
5 Assessment results of trainees	26 Peer review of the medical team
6 Audit	27 Personal invigoration
7 Changes in person specification	28 Protection from successful litigation
8 Changing practice	29 Recruitment of medical staff
9 Clinical effectiveness	30 Reduction in burn-out and early retirement
10 CPD credit points	31 Referrals to the doctor
11 Collaborative assessment	32 Remunerative benefit: discretionary points, merit awards, etc.
12 Confidence levels	33 Reporting back to colleagues
13 Corporate image	34 Reputation as trainer
14 Decreasing professional isolation	35 Research
15 'Don't know' factor	36 Risk management
16 Educational culture	37 Self-assessment
17 Educational record and logbooks	38 Time-efficient working
18 Effects on the team	39 Video assessment
19 Enhancing practice	40 Video-stimulated recall
20 Learning diaries	41 Written reports
21 Learning portfolios	

Moving on

The advent of clinical governance affects every aspect of the management and delivery of healthcare. It demands changes in infrastructure and process. With regard to CPD, the role of GP tutors, for example, and the relationship between primary care groups and the Directors of Postgraduate General Practice Education will require consideration. There are many strands to be interwoven and roles to be coordinated. Some of these can be resolved at a regional or local level but other issues can only be resolved at a national level – primary among these is the question of how GPs' Postgraduate Education Allowance (PGEA) might work in relation to managed CPD.

Discussions on this point will need to address organisation and management issues, funding streams and processes. A change of focus is required so that the successful implementation of well-managed CPD, with all its features as described here, is recognised by the funding arrangements. A funding system which implies that simple attendance at an educational event is good enough regardless of need, quality or benefit to practitioner or practice will no longer be professionally acceptable. Of course, such events will still feature in the educational activities of GPs – there is nothing in managed CPD that precludes the doctor from learning in any particular way – but the educational event itself will no longer be the sole feature of education. Instead, that event will become part of a process of learning that starts with practice and returns to practice. It is that process, fundamental to clinical governance, which funding arrangements must now recognise.

Practical points

> The term CPD is preferred to CME – it encompasses a broader content of learning and covers all professional groups.
>
> - CPD is central to the implementation of clinical governance.
> - CPD should be managed locally – at the primary care team level.
> - PPDPs should incorporate PDPs for the whole team.
> - The method used to learn is not as important as the process of assessing educational needs beforehand, and reinforcing and disseminating the learning afterwards.
> - For CPD to be effective it is vital to get the process right.

References

1 Department of Health (1998) *A First Class Service: quality in the new NHS*. Health Service Circular: HSC(98)113. Department of Health, London.

2 Department of Health (1998) *A Review of Continuing Professional Development in General Practice. A Report by the Chief Medical Officer*. Department of Health, London.

3 Grant J and Stanton F (1998) *The Effectiveness of Continuing Professional Development. A Report for the Chief Medical Officer's Review of Continuing Professional Development in General Practice* (2e). Joint Centre for Education in Medicine, London.

4 Davis DA, Thomson MA, Oxman AD and Haynes B (1995) Changing physician performance: a systematic review of the effect of continuing medical education strategies. *JAMA*. **247**: 700–5.

5 Grant J, Chambers E and Jackson G (1999) *The Good CPD Guide*. Reed Healthcare Publishing, Sutton.

6 Knowles N (1990) *The Adult Learner: a neglected species* (4e). Gulf Publishing Co, Houston, TX.

7 Ramsey PG, Carline JD, Inui TS, Larson EB, LoGerfo JP and Weinrich MD (1989) Predictive validity of certification by the American Board of Internal Medicine. *Annals of Internal Medicine*. **110**: 719–26.

8 Paget NS, Newble DI, Saunders NS and Du J (1996) Physician assessment pilot study for the Royal Australasian College of Physicians. *Journal of Continuing Education in the Health Professions*. **16**: 103–11.

CHAPTER THIRTEEN

Developing leaders

Jamie Harrison

Leadership remains the most studied and least understood topic in all the social sciences

Warren Bennis

This chapter explores how to develop leaders, and leadership, in primary care. In a time of change, the complementary roles of leadership and management are highlighted, and a pattern of servant leadership is suggested for the future.

Introduction

Primary care has not always been good at developing leaders. Certainly, within traditional general practice, the rule was that GPs led the organisation, with the doctor with the greatest seniority controlling the GPs – whether or not that individual was a skilled leader.

Hence, team leadership was based purely on length of clinical experience (or time served in the practice), rather than on ability to lead. More recently, this hierarchical approach has been challenged by the introduction of executive partners and profession-ally trained practice managers into local practices, and by health authority managers working alongside GPs within commissioning groups and primary care groups.

Nevertheless, many GPs are cautious about being directed in how to do their work. Equally, they remain suspicious of those who seek to lead them. Partly this reflects the fact that, historically, GPs have valued their independence, individualism and relative lack of accountability. As a result, they have found it difficult to find a consensus in formulating policy matters, not least in how to respond to government's proposed contractual changes, notably in 1990.

This inability to find a common mind on matters of policy, in tandem with an unwillingness to carry out concerted action, suggests that, were they proverbial horses, GPs would never allow themselves to be led to water, and certainly not agree to drink.

Others in primary care may not be so fiercely individualistic, but they can be hampered by training and employment cultures which suppress initiative and independent thinking. Again, this is changing, as nurses, managers and those professionals allied to medicine are allowed to develop as independent practitioners, as well as leaders of uniprofessional teams.

The role of clinical governance in this area is complex. Whilst seeking to balance a proper desire for greater professional freedom, there is a need for corporate accountability within multiprofessional primary care teams. And the world of primary care itself is changing rapidly. Teams will need good leadership if they are to cope with the rate of change, which, if anything, is accelerating.

What is leadership?

The new quality agenda[1] puts added pressure on primary care teams who have, for whatever reason, failed to move with the times. Yet all practices and practitioners can do better. Clinical governance is suggested as the means by which everyone in primary care will improve. But, within the clinical governance agenda, it is worth asking what will drive the various components described. Is effective leadership the necessary first mechanism, which will initially trigger, and then guide and encourage, the full set of governance mechanisms? For, indeed, without leadership, will clinical governance get off the ground at all?

Professor John Kotter, from the Harvard Business School, reminds us that leadership is vital during times of change, and that leadership is different from management:

> *Management is about coping with complexity ... Leadership, by contrast, is about coping with change ... More change demands more leadership.*[2]

So primary care must come to accept that, in a rapidly changing environment, effective leadership will be increasingly necessary, and that better management, on its own, is insufficient to deal with the new quality agenda. For leadership is the means by which the quality agenda can be driven forward, leaving it to management to solve the problems created in its wake (*see* Box 13.1) And we must never lose sight of the fact that 'leadership complements management; it doesn't replace it'.[2]

For Kotter, effective leaders should have the following attributes:

- vision, with the ability to formulate strategies
- ready access to a reservoir of support mechanisms, with which to respond to changing situations for themselves and others
- the ability or charisma to increase motivation and build a team or teams.

But how is leadership to be developed; what makes a good leader?

Box 13.1: Differences between leadership and management

Leadership	*Management*
Develops strategy	Puts strategy into practice
Copes with change	Copes with complexity
Creates the team	Maintains the team
Increases motivation and inspires	Monitors and solves problems

---

How to develop as a leader

Ken Jarrold is clear that we learn about leadership from the example of others – through reading literature, hearing stories, seeing events in the news, and by reflecting on our own experience of leadership, and leaders, within the NHS. For him, leadership is about service:

> *If leadership is about showing the way, about knowing what to do next, about the courage to stand against, about giving people space, how do you do it? You lead by serving.*[3]

He goes on to offer five steps to those who are willing to grow as servant leaders:

- *learn to listen*: to questions and requests for advice; for information, experience, wisdom and knowledge
- *keep thinking*: sort information; analyse and grapple with issues
- *foster sound judgement*: evaluate the situation; decide what is right
- *be clear*: explain your analysis and decision; people and organisations require clarity
- *be courageous*: not to be confused with arrogance; servant leaders need humility, but they also need courage – 'the power to stand against' (Peter Ackroyd).

For Jarrold, the last word in this area goes to David Wilkinson and Elaine Applebee, where the emphasis, for them, is on the need for courage in leadership, rather than simply charisma:

> *Leaders communicate more by what they do, champion and support, than by what they say. They are able to substantially increase the stock of leadership across the system, generating a wide commitment to act, learn and take risks. It is feedback from this that in turn sustains effective leaders. It is important that leaders find their own styles, and can act with a range of styles contingent upon the situation. Above all, they need to be able to live and work with paradox, dilemmas and uncertainty – both their own and others.*[4]

Yet leaders must find ways in which to engage with those they are called upon to lead. The type of leadership style they adopt will profoundly influence their relationship with a team or organisation, and hence play a major role in the effectiveness of the whole enterprise.

Leadership styles

Leadership style can range from authoritarian to democratic, to *laissez-faire*. In the authoritarian, the leader makes the decisions; in the democratic, the group decides by majority vote; in the *laissez-faire*, the leader allows individuals to decide for themselves, or not to decide at all – depending on how the team or organisation feels at the time.[5]

How leaders lead depends on context, occasion and their personal beliefs about leadership. The most dominant of these is the leader's own personal value system. Leaders who value status and position will resent any attempts to undermine their authority and power. Leaders who see themselves as servants will not.

Equally, within teams, there will be expectations of how the leader should lead. If a team expects firm leadership, its members may block the leader's attempts to encourage participation in decision-making – after all, that's the leader's job. Young teams, and newly formulated organisations such as primary care group boards and clinical governance sub-groups, may find their members drawn from a wide range of professional and other backgrounds. Care will be needed initially to give such groupings direction. In a new situation, it is unwise to try to use highly participative approaches too soon.

And tailoring leadership style to the context is important. However democratic the clinical team, during a cardiac arrest it is inappropriate to take a vote on the dose of adrenaline to be administered. Someone needs to take charge and give the orders. Once the emergency has passed, there will be time to reflect together on the next course of action.

The more mature the team and its leader, the more flexible and innovative can be the leadership, moving easily between directive, democratic and easy-going styles, as and when the situation demands. Figure 13.1 highlights the various hierarchies of leadership

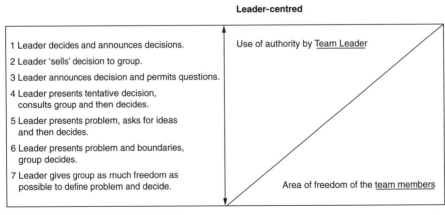

Figure 13.1   Leadership styles (based on the Tannenbaum Schmidt model[5]).

observed in practice within organisations, with the relative degree of power exercised by leader and team member shown on the right of the figure.

David Cormack concludes with five general principles in regard to leadership style:

- there is probably no single right style of leader behaviour
- effective leaders base their behaviour on the context in which they find themselves
- effective leaders can modify their leadership style to fit the demands of the situation
- team members are confused and frustrated when leaders behave differently from how they expect their leader to lead
- effective leaders of mature teams operate as near to the group-centred end of the continuum of power sharing as is possible in any one situation.

Leaders may find it helpful to reflect on their own preferred leadership style. Whatever that may be, the goal of leadership remains the same – to achieve results, success in the team or organisation's chosen field. For primary care, that means meeting the needs of patients in an accessible, comprehensive, coordinated and continuing way.

Leadership in primary care

Leaders in primary care work at the sharp end of the health service, being required not only to manage change, but to lead it. This requires the ability to shape, share and articulate vision and strategy, excellent communication skills, drive and enthusiasm, political awareness and the ability to motivate and support others. As Tim van Zwanenberg puts it, such leaders:

> must rise above parochial and professional vested interests. Leadership is neither wholly an innate quality nor wholly a learned skill. Some have an aptitude to become leaders and they need opportunities to develop the appropriate skills.[6]

The challenge to primary care is how to identify, train and nurture such leaders. Already, primary care group clinical governance leads have articulated their desire for support in this area (*see* Box 13.2).

Clinical governance leads in primary care groups obviously feel the need to develop skills in both management and leadership, notably in strategic thinking, motivation, team leadership and change management. Interviews with GPs produced similar results, with a comment that 'there was nothing in general practitioner training about team development or leadership, and that this was a considerable omission in their development which needed to be addressed.'[7]

Strategic thinking

Since the function of leadership is to produce change, setting the direction of that change is fundamental. Setting direction is not the same as planning, or even long-term planning,

---

Box 13.2:   Development needs identified by primary care group clinical governance leads[7]

- strategic thinking   ⎫
- motivation   ⎪
- team leadership   ⎬   LEADERSHIP SKILLS
- change management   ⎭

- negotiation

- the development of systems for measuring care   ⎫
- dissemination   ⎪
- marketing   ⎬   MANAGEMENT SKILLS
- risk management   ⎭

---

although the two are often confused. For planning is a management process, deductive in nature and designed to produce orderly results, not change.

> *Setting a direction is more inductive. Leaders gather a broad range of data and look for patterns, relationships, and linkages that help explain things. What's more, the direction-setting aspect of leadership does not produce plans; it creates vision and strategies.*[2]

Kotter goes on to develop the idea of how to develop a strategy:

> *Nor do visions and strategies have to be brilliantly innovative; in fact, some of the best are not. Effective (business) visions regularly have an almost mundane quality, usually consisting of ideas that are already well known. The particular combination of the ideas may be new, but sometimes even that is not the case.*

In the context of primary care, there are plenty of good ideas, innovations and practical strategies already in use somewhere in the UK. There is no need to reinvent the wheel. What is crucial is to become aware of this rich seam of options, and to harness the most useful and appropriate to inform local strategies. This process must also take into account the needs of the stake holders – health authorities, primary care staff and patients.

Charles Handy describes the characteristics necessary for a strategy or vision to be effective, making the point that 'a leader shapes and shares a vision which gives point to the work of others'[8] (*see* Box 13.3).

Motivation

Motivation comes from within, the feelings and attitudes experienced in response to basic needs. Whatever the popular view, you cannot, in fact, 'motivate' someone else. You can, however, create situations in which they, or others, will be motivated.

Box 13.3:   Characteristics of an effective vision or strategy

- must be different
- must make sense to others
- must stretch people's imagination but be achievable
- must be understandable
- must be lived by the leader
- must be believed in, and enacted, by the whole team

After Handy.[8]

The work of Abraham Maslow[9] describes five basic human needs: to have, to be, to do, to love and to grow. His analysis contains the notion of a hierarchy of needs, in that individuals vary in both their perceived 'basic' needs and in what motivates them beyond their minimum requirements for survival.

The leader's role is to provide an environment in which people are motivated – where team members are able to satisfy their needs whilst also doing what the team requires of them. This is shown in Figure 13.2.

Some people are motivated by nice working conditions, extra holidays and financial reward; others by the knowledge that they are doing a good job, have status in the team and are valued. The art of the team leader in primary care is to identify what motivates each individual team member, creating the right atmosphere, opportunities and incentives for that person to develop.

Team leadership

Team leadership is closely allied to creating a work environment which helps individuals to be motivated and to perform well. Any one individual's current needs will change from time to time, as their domestic circumstances and work contexts alter. New team members will first need to gain acceptance within the team. As they become established, they will need new challenges and greater responsibility. Leaders need to facilitate this.

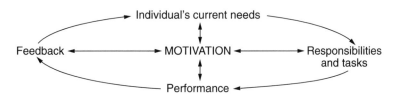

Figure 13.2   A model of motivation.

The role and effectiveness of each member will need regular clarification if stagnation and confusion are to be avoided. The team leader has the responsibility to ensure that all team members are clear about their respective roles within the organisation, how they fit in with colleagues, what the overall strategy is and how they are performing, both individually and as a unit. This involves leaders setting targets and giving team members properly resourced opportunities to perform, with good feedback and formal appraisal.

It goes without saying that good communication is essential if effective leadership is to thrive. Leaders in primary care need to trust their team members, act with integrity, tell the truth, welcome constructive comment and criticism, and lead by example. Such leaders will need to be directive on occasions, take responsibility and make hard decisions when necessary.

Change management

Change is a natural process, although recently the health service seems to have had more than its fair share. For many in primary care, change is difficult. And as we have already noted, leadership is about coping with change; it must therefore be about helping to manage the changes thrust upon colleagues and team members.

Change occurs for a number of reasons. In primary care, change can result from:

- national initiatives and the imposition of new NHS frameworks, e.g. clinical governance
- the formation of new local organisational structures, e.g. primary care groups
- changes to primary care team personnel, e.g. one health visitor leaves and is replaced by another
- changes to the team's character, e.g. the team grows tired and stale
- new demands on the team's services, e.g. added work from early hospital discharges.

All these changes must be managed; that is to say, they must be handled in such a way that moves the team forward in pursuit of its purposes. To do so, leaders must continue to review strategy, resource allocation, methods of monitoring and workload. Promoting communication, team member training, learning from experience and learning from others in a similar situation would also seem to be essential.

Leadership in primary care groups and primary care teams

Primary care groups

By now, primary care groups should have in post their board chairs, chief executives and clinical governance leads. By training and profession, chairs will most likely be doctors, chief executives, managers and governance leads taken from a mix of nursing and medical backgrounds. Their capacity to develop as leaders depends on: their innate ability; a commitment to the leadership task; appropriate training; the support and encouragement of colleagues; and being provided with adequate time, personnel and financial resources.

The roles of chair and chief executive are obviously different, although both require leadership skills. The primary care group itself is a federation of organisations, and as such demands a different type of leadership when compared with a single organisational structure. Negotiation will be important, as well as clarity of strategic thinking and effective communication.

The framework for the first year of clinical governance includes establishing leadership in primary care groups (*see* Table 1.2, p. 7 for a detailed commentary).[10] The essential issues for leaders are those of inclusivity, openness, clarity, cooperation, commitment, communication and accountability. Lay board members have a key role to play in reviewing the effectiveness of such leadership, and in acting as a bridge for leaders to the wider community.

Primary care group clinical governance leads will need both to build a team within their governance sub-groups and to draw together the governance leads within the individual primary care teams. This will require skill in diplomacy, a clear strategy and the ability to listen. Being realistic about what is achievable, allied to creating an environment which motivates others, would also appear to be necessary.

In subsequent years, primary care groups will need to develop leadership that: learns from its own experiences; reflects on the wisdom of others; identifies new leaders locally; thinks strategically, especially about primary care trust formation; and builds up and develops the infrastructure of primary care. It might be worth remembering Tim van Zwanenberg's key strategic themes for tomorrow's GP, themes which have validity for all in primary care (*see* Box 13.4).

Box 13.4:   Strategic themes for primary care[6]

Leadership
- vision
- communication skills
- motivating others
- above vested interests

Scholarship
- learning valued
- research and teaching
- higher qualifications

Fellowship
- mutual support
- flexible careers
- mentoring

Primary care teams

Leadership within primary care teams will continue to be carried out predominantly by doctors. This reflects a combination of their status, ownership of practice premises and the fact that many primary care staff are currently employees of GP partnerships.

However, things are changing. Nurse leadership within Primary Care Act pilot schemes and the appointment of nurses as primary care group clinical governance leads points one way for the future. There is no reason why practice nurses, district nurses or health visitors should not be primary care team governance leads. Indeed, this is already happening.

Yet most clearly, there needs to be the creation of a culture of leadership within practices and primary care teams. Sadly, the on-the-job experiences of many people actually seem to undermine their development as leaders. Recruiting those with leadership potential is one step.

Another is to manage the career and work patterns of established team members, by creating challenging opportunities, allowing exposure to a wide range of leaders and contexts, and by broadening experience, both within and beyond the health service, through sabbaticals, both home and abroad, secondment to non-NHS organisations and involvement in networking ventures such as Common Purpose.

These wide experiences teach people about life, how others lead, how society operates and how patients think in the world outside the NHS. More importantly, they also teach people in primary care teams something about both the difficulty of leadership and its potential for producing change.

Encouraging tomorrow's leaders in primary care

Leadership in primary care is at a crossroads. As more is asked of primary care, by government, patients, managers and clinical staff, exciting new possibilities present themselves. As Ken Jarrold comments:

> *We need to recognize and encourage the leaders in primary care. The most able leaders in primary care sustain both local communities and the NHS. The most successful leaders of primary care groups will have a strong claim to leadership in the NHS.*[3]

Can primary care rise to the challenge? Will the leaders of primary care – to be found within primary care groups, primary care teams, uniprofessional local organisations (LMC, RCN, RCGP and their equivalents), undergraduate and postgraduate university departments, and health authority primary care directorates – grasp the opportunities offered by the new quality agenda? If so, they must recognise that there are other leaders within the NHS who demand their respect, with whom they can work and from whom they can learn (*see* Box 13.5).

Box 13.5:   Other leaders in the NHS

- patient and carer leaders
- public leaders (local communities)
- political leaders
- NHS trade union leaders
- NHS management leaders
- secondary care leaders

After Jarrold.[3]

Identifying and training tomorrow's leaders is an on-going task, which will need imagination, resources (from both inside and outside the NHS) and time. And such leaders must not lose sight of the prime purpose of primary care, which is to respond appropriately to the needs of patients and their carers. For those working in primary care in the NHS – an organisation funded by taxation, with its ethos firmly that of public service – it may be wise to remember how health service leaders differ from senior managers in strictly commercial ventures, such as a public limited company (plc), and respond accordingly (*see* Box 13.6).

Developing leaders in primary care will continue to be demanding and rewarding. To be truly effective, leaders will need both to receive the title 'leader' from their organ-isation and to earn the right to lead, by their example. And no leader will gain the following of a team without first showing and experiencing a personal commitment to the team itself, its individual members and the task that is set before it – all lived out in the spirit of service:

> *the leader must know that he is most deeply committed to his followers, most heavily laden with responsibility towards the orders of life, in fact quite simply a servant.*[11]

Ultimately, primary care must create leaders, and leadership, if it is to develop and change how its teams and organisations function, thereby bringing benefit to all – patients, clinicians and managers alike. Where a corporate culture exists that values

---

Box 13.6:   Differences between public and private sector leaders

NHS leaders	*Managing directors (plc)*
Value diversity of style across teams	Impose corporate culture
Non-profit ethos	Profit maximisation
Respect and care for all equally	Target specific consumer groups
De-centralise power (subsidiarity)	Centralise decision-making
End – healthy people	*End* – healthy profit

---

effective, servant leadership, and strives to maintain and further such leadership, the organisation concerned truly flourishes.

Developing such a culture is the work of a leader. Within the complexity of contemporary primary care, that would seem to be an essential task. Indeed, institutionalising a leadership-centred culture could be seen as the ultimate act of leadership.

Practical points

- Leadership is about creating and coping with change.
- Management is about coping with complexity.
- Leadership is required to get clinical governance off the ground; management to implement its many components.
- Leaders adopt different styles – the best leaders using the style apropriate for the situation.
- In primary care the style of servant-leader may allow both the formulation of strategy and the creation of an environnment in which team members are motivated.
- There is a need to identify and nurture primary care leaders of the future.

References

1   Department of Health (1998) *A First Class Service: quality in the new NHS*. Health Service Circular: HSC(98)113. Department of Health, London.

2   Kotter JP (1999) *What Leaders Really Do*. Harvard Business Review Books, Cambridge, MA.

3   Jarrold K (1998) Servants and leaders: leadership in the NHS. In: *York Syposium on Health – a report of the fourth symposium held at the University of York 30 July 1998*. Department of Health Studies, University of York.

4   Wilkinson D and Applebee E (1999) *Implementing Holistic Government – joined up action on the ground*. The Policy Press, University of Bristol.

5   Cormack D (1987) *Team Spirit. People Working with People*. MARC Europe, Bromley. For a more detailed analysis of leadership styles, Schein EH (1988) *Organizational Psychology*. Prentice-Hall, Englewood Cliffs, NJ.

6   Van Zwanenberg T (1998) GP Tomorrow. In: J Harrison and T van Zwanenberg (eds) *GP Tomorrow*. Radcliffe Medical Press, Oxford.

7   Firth-Cozens J (1999) *Report on clinical governance development needs in health service staff*. University of Northumbria, Newcastle.

8   Handy C (1991) *The Age of Unreason*. Arrow Business Books, London.

9   Maslow A (1954) *Motivation and Personality.* Harper and Row, New York.

10   Department of Health (1999) *Clinical Governance: quality in the new NHS.* Department of Health, London.

11   Bonhoeffer D (1965) *No Rusty Swords. Letters, Lectures and Notes 1928–1936.* Collins, London.

PART 3

Exploring the future

CHAPTER FOURTEEN

Educating the coming generation

John Spencer

Medical education is a reflection of medical practice; it is not the education that will change the practitioners, but reformed practice that will redesign medical education.

George Silver (1983)

This chapter explains how the clinical governance agenda is already present within the undergraduate and training curriculum. It highlights the need to embody clinical governance in all aspects of the student's experience and introduces the concept of curricular governance.

The background

It is self-evident that health professions in training should be prepared for the challenges of future practice, as far, that is, as such challenges can be anticipated. Indeed, much has been written about the need to ensure that all basic professional training takes account of both the emerging role of the doctor- or nurse-to-be and of the realities of everyday practice, and, that such education is relevant to the changing needs and expectations of society.[1,2]

Equally, implementing clinical governance looks likely to be one of the major challenges facing healthcare professionals in the UK for the foreseeable future. Such a task has important implications for those involved in the basic education of doctors, nurses and other professions allied to medicine. Although, in the various policy documents, much has been written about the educational implications of clinical governance for *established* practitioners, conspicuous by their absence are any substantive references to the implications for the basic education of health professionals. When the issue *is* mentioned, universities are criticised for having neither 'adopted the new quality agenda' nor helped learners develop the skills of 'knowledge management'.[3]

In reality, undergraduate education in most medical schools in the UK has undergone major change in the 1990s, largely in response to, and guided by, the recommendations of the GMC in its influential document *Tomorrow's Doctors*.[4] This identified the need to produce doctors whose attitude to both medicine and learning would equip them for lifelong professional careers. Hence, where lifelong learning becomes the main aim of the undergraduate course, what is required, among other things, is a reduction in the factual burden of curricula, and the promotion of the capacity for self-education, evaluation of evidence and critical thinking (*see* Box 14.1). Within a culture of lifelong learning must also come the ability to forget, thereby putting aside ways of thinking and acting that have become outmoded.

Implicit in these recommendations, and made explicit in subsequent GMC publications such as *Good Medical Practice*,[5] was the nature of the contract between the medical profession and society. Issues such as the need for high moral and ethical standards, the importance of keeping up-to-date, the duty to protect all patients and the importance of working in teams are all highlighted.

A similar change has taken place in nurse education in the last decade.[6]

Box 14.1: Principal recommendations for change in undergraduate medical education

- Reduction of factual burden.
- Promotion of learning through curiosity, exploration of knowledge and critical evaluation of evidence.
- Inculcation of 'attitudes of mind and of behaviour that befit a doctor'.
- Greater emphasis on acquisition of skills, adequately supervised and rigorously assessed.
- Definition of a 'core curriculum', encompassing essential knowledge, skills and attitudes.
- Augmentation of core with a series of 'special study modules', allowing students to study in depth topics of interest to them, to provide insights into scientific method, and to 'engender an approach to medicine that is questioning and self-critical'.
- Increased emphasis on communication skills and other aspects of clinical method.
- Greater emphasis on the theme of public health medicine.
- Response to changing patterns of healthcare, in particular increased experience in the community and primary care.
- Learning systems informed by modern educational theory.
- Establishment of effective supervisory structures.

From *Tomorrow's Doctors*.[4]

Implications for the education of healthcare practitioners

A recent editorial highlighted the implications of clinical governance for medical education.[7] It concerned itself as much with the education of nurses, and other healthcare professionals, as with the education of doctors (*see* Box 14.2).

Box 14.2:   Key issues for medical educators in relation to clinical governance

- Ensure the acquisition of requisite skills and understanding.
- Introduce the concept of clinical governance early.
- Apply the principles of clinical governance to educational activities.
- Promote the values that underpin clinical governance.

From Morrison and Buckley.[7]

First, practitioners need to acquire the necessary understanding and skills if they are to utilise such tools as clinical audit, critical appraisal and risk assessment. Second, the concept of clinical governance should be introduced to learners from the beginning, and then remain as a continuous theme in curricula. Third, educators must be prepared to practice what they preach, and to apply the principles of clinical governance to their own educational activities. Finally, and perhaps most important of all, is the need to promote the values that underpin the concept of clinical governance.

To this list of issues could also be added the need to develop appropriate skills and attitudes in relation to teamwork, and the ability to use the principles of management effectively.

The current situation

Gaining understanding and learning skills

Some of the component activities of clinical governance are already being addressed in undergraduate curricula and pre-registration courses, albeit often delivered as 'stand alone' courses developed by enthusiasts, and not necessarily integrated into the curriculum. In many ways, this mirrors the situation in practice at the time of writing.[8] For example, innovative models for teaching and learning about clinical audit have been described, such as where medical students undertake audit projects during clinical attachments in general practice. These brief courses are generally highly valued by students and involvement in them also appears to be beneficial for both GP tutors and patients alike.[9,10]

Models, and methods, are available for teaching the skills of critical appraisal and evidence-based medicine,[11] and for learning about medical informatics, which encompasses a broad range of topics such as clinical information systems, medical record-keeping, decision-making and decision support, and the use of guidelines.[12]

Teaching and learning about ethics and medical aspects of law is now well established in many curricula, often taught alongside communication skills,[13] and recommendations have been made about a 'core' curriculum for the content of such courses.[14] With ethics and the law come moral questions about life and death, rationing and being professionals in today's world. Grounding all such learning, as far as possible, in practice, rather than in theory, and on concrete examples (ideally real cases based on the experiences of the learners) is vital – promoting relevance, fostering integration of knowledge and motivating learners.[15]

Teamworking

Effective teamworking is said to promote clinical governance. Interprofessional education, whereby students from different professional backgrounds in health and social care spend time learning together, is seen as one way whereby teamworking skills might be developed.[16] However, although a national survey in the UK in 1996 by the Centre for the Advancement of Inter-professional Education showed that initiatives in interprofessional education were 'wide ranging, varied, increasing, evolving and developing',[17] there were relatively few reported at undergraduate level, and even fewer involving the medical profession. Furthermore, systematic reviews have shown that simple descriptions of courses are more common in the literature than any evidence of their effectiveness, and that evaluations of benefits beyond the short term have been marred by methodological problems.[18]

Nonetheless, there have been studies of interprofessional education (in both the UK and elsewhere) that have demonstrated increased mutual understanding, and respect, through the identification of 'common values, knowledge, and skills across professions and work settings and creating a shared philosophy of care',[19] with more positive attitudes towards the importance of multidisciplinary teamwork and communication resulting.[18] Despite the lack of evidence so far, intuitively it seems the right thing to encourage shared learning, with the potential to influence the development of the practitioners of the new century, for whom new ways of working together are an inevitability. Some of the benefits claimed for effective interprofessional education are shown in Box 14.3.

Box 14.3:   Principles of effective interprofessional education

- Works to improve the quality of care.
- Focuses on the needs of service users and carers.
- Involves service users and carers.
- Promotes interprofessional collaboration.
- Encourages professions to learn with, from and about one another.
- Enhances practice within professions.
- Respects the integrity and contribution of each profession.
- Increases professional satisfaction.

From Barr and Waterton.[17]

Introducing the concept of clinical governance systematically

The increased emphasis in curricula on skills acquisition, 'knowledge management',[3] ethical reasoning and the promotion of lifelong learning, as well as on pastoral and personal development, has led to the development in some medical schools of courses which draw such themes together into a coherent curricular structure. This process starts early, and runs through the whole curriculum, interweaving, where appropriate, with teaching and learning in the basic and clinical sciences. Such integration provides an ideal vehicle for introducing concepts of clinical governance. At the same time, the so-called 'man in society'-type courses[4] (which usually cover human development, aspects of sociology and psychology relevant to health, illness and disease, and so on) are also being introduced by many medical schools, alongside an increased emphasis on public health medicine.

An example from Newcastle's new curriculum is shown in Box 14.4. This 'Personal and Professional Development Strand' is introduced in the first week of the medical course, and is set in the context of the GMC's guidelines for good medical practice[5] and core professional values.[20]

A broad view of communication skills is taken, encompassing doctor–patient and intraprofessional communication, written and presentation skills, electronic communication, and group and teamworking skills.

'Methods of inquiry' covers a wide range of skills related to 'knowledge management', including critical appraisal and evidence-based medicine, information technology and library skills, research methods and statistics, and decision-making.

'Context of care' emphasises that healthcare is delivered in a multiplicity of settings, by a wide variety of healthcare professionals, each professional group with its own internal 'culture'. That culture influences the organisation of teams, relationships and even the way care is ultimately delivered. Professional codes of practice are explored alongside basic principles in the 'ethics' component.

Box 14.4:   The 'Personal and Professional Development Strand' at Newcastle Medical School

School
- Starts in first year and runs as a vertical theme throughout the five-year curriculum.
- Integrates with teaching and learning in basic and clinical sciences.
- Where appropriate is assessed.

Themes
- communication skills
- clinical skills
- ethics
- methods of inquiry
- clinical reasoning
- context of care
- self-care (including study skills support and pastoral support)

The 'self-care' theme addresses personal development through both academic and pastoral support. This area has been somewhat neglected in medical education in the past. In the light of the high levels of stress and of maladaptive behaviours reported by medical students,[21] and the influence this might have on subsequent morale and performance, this neglect needs to be addressed.

Newcastle's 'medicine in society' course also starts in week one, and covers a number of areas relevant to clinical governance, such as working in groups, the relationship between the profession and the community it serves, making sense of data (both quantitative and qualitative) and aspects of population medicine.

The development of reflective abilities is highly pertinent to clinical governance. Promotion of reflective practice, and of self-awareness, is already well developed in nurse education,[22] and is an emerging theme in undergraduate medical curricula.[23]

Practising what we preach – curricular governance

In parallel with the development and implementation of new courses in medical schools, there has been something of a cultural change in the way curricula are managed. This has come about partly as a response to increasing concern about quality issues, with demands for greater accountability, and partly as an inevitable consequence of moving towards more innovative educational approaches. Curriculum design, implementation and management have become more strategic, underpinned by recognition of the fact that underlying systems are as important as course content, in the delivery of high-quality teaching and learning.

Curriculum governance has been described as 'a system through which teaching institutions and individual teachers are accountable for continuously improving the quality of their course and safeguarding high standards of teaching by creating an environment in which excellence in teaching and learning will flourish' (J Bligh, personal communication), and, as with its clinical counterpart, it resonates with corporate governance. Essential components of curriculum governance must therefore include strong and transparent management systems, rigorous and systematic evaluation of courses, and staff development.[24,25]

Student involvement is a key element of curriculum governance, and plays an important part in the process of quality management and enhancement. Here students assume a role equivalent to that of patients in the context of clinical governance, and for them this involvement creates a sense of ownership and partnership, and may even improve motivation.[26,27] Some medical schools have been particularly innovative in involving students in the curriculum. For example, Liverpool not only has student membership of all course committees, but, in addition, has a student parliament in which elected student members meet on a regular basis to discuss the problems and solutions.[28]

Promoting appropriate values

Clinical governance is as much about an attitude of mind as it is about skills and systems. Inculcation of appropriate professional attitudes and values has assumed prominence in the recommendations of the bodies governing basic and pre-registration education of healthcare professionals. For example, the attitudinal objectives of *Tomorrow's Doctors* are shown in Box 14.5, all of which, to a greater or lesser degree, have some relevance to learning about clinical governance.

Box 14.5:   The GMC's attitudinal objectives for undergraduate curricula

* Respect for patients and colleagues that encompasses, without prejudice, diversity of background and opportunity, language, culture and way of life.
* The recognition of patients' rights in all respects, and particularly in regard to confidentiality and informed consent.
* Approaches to learning that are based on curiosity and the exploration of knowledge rather than on its passive acquisition, and that will be retained throughout professional life.
* Ability to cope with uncertainty.
* Awareness of the moral and ethical responsibilities involved in individual patient care and in the provision of care to populations; such awareness must be developed early in the course.

Box 14.5:   cont

- Awareness of the need to ensure that the highest possible quality of patient care must always be provided.
- Development of the capacity for self-audit and for participation in the peer review process.
- Awareness of personal limitations, a willingness to seek help when necessary and ability to work effectively as a member of a team.
- Willingness to use his or her professional capabilities to contribute to community as well as to individual patient welfare by the practice of preventive medicine and the encouragement of health promotion.
- Ability to adapt to change.
- Awareness of the need for continuing professional development allied to the process of continuing medical education, in order to ensure that high levels of clinical competence and knowledge are maintained.
- Acceptance of the responsibility to contribute as far as possible to the advancement of medical knowledge in order to benefit medical practice and further improve the quality of patient care.

From *Tomorrow's Doctors*.[4]

The increased emphasis in many curricula on communication skills may also help students adopt a clinical method that is more patient-centred than the traditional paternalistic approach – one that fosters a genuine partnership between healthcare professional and patient.[29]

Facilitating the development of attitudes is one thing. However, if the acquisition of such attitudes is not assessed in some way, it will not be given a high priority by students. Similarly, if students do not see clinical governance 'in action' during their clinical attachments, the impact of the teaching and learning will be diluted considerably. The concept of the 'hidden curriculum' is useful in this context. A curriculum can be thought of as comprising three elements: 'the curriculum on paper' (what is intended or hoped the course will achieve); 'the curriculum in action' (what is delivered on the day); and 'the curriculum the student experiences'. The latter can be very different, both from what is intended and what actually happens.[15] The relationship between these three curricula is shown in Figure 14.1.

That part of the curriculum that is neither explicitly intended nor formally taught is known as the 'hidden curriculum'. This was first described in the context of primary school education,[30] but is a potent force in all educational settings and forms a large part of a student's learning experience. It is effectively a 'parallel' curriculum through which students learn the values, norms and expectations of an educational environment. It can be a more powerful influence than teachers might imagine, for example in the socialisation of students, or in determining whether students decide to study

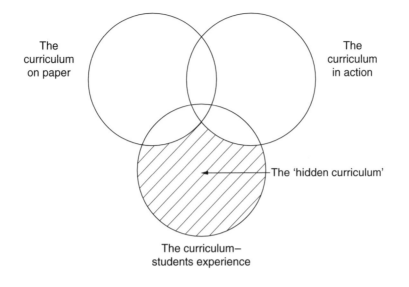

The curriculum on paper

The curriculum in action

The 'hidden curriculum'

The curriculum—
students experience

Figure 14.1 The three curricula and the hidden curriculum.

a subject based on whether it is assessed. One cannot overestimate the effect assessment has in driving learning, influencing both *what* students learn and *how* they learn it.

Historically, assessment has often been merely an add-on extra, but now it is increasingly assuming its rightful role as a crucial component of curriculum design. It is therefore important, in respect of teaching and learning about clinical governance, to ensure that whatever relevant areas can be appropriately assessed actually *are* assessed. This may require new ways of thinking about assessment, for example as a process that is formative and not simply a stressful hazard to be negotiated on the way to graduation. Assessing some of these areas of learning will also require the use of more innovative methods.

The role of primary care in the basic education of healthcare professionals

One trend that has been gathering momentum in healthcare education in recent years is the move to deliver more basic teaching and learning in the community. In the context of medical education in the UK this has usually meant more experience in general practice, although, increasingly, a wider view of the 'community' is being taken.[18,31]

Besides learning specifically about the discipline of general practice, doctors in training can benefit by:

- learning about health, disease and disability in its social context, and about the environmental and social determinants of disease
- seeing the full range of presentation of health problems
- having opportunities to learn basic clinical and communication skills on relatively well patients
- experiencing a more holistic approach to patient care
- better integration of knowledge and understanding
- experiencing continuity of care
- learning to manage uncertainty and to handle ambiguity
- seeing multidisciplinary teamwork in action.

It has been argued that, in many ways, primary care is the ideal setting for educating 'tomorrow's doctors', where critical reasoning, self-awareness and reflectiveness, and the ability to handle uncertainty – all highly pertinent in the context of clinical governance – can be fostered.[32]

Making it happen – curricular change

Implementing curricular change is difficult. Models for managing innovation in medical education have been outlined,[33] a process that starts with the identification of potential barriers. One key barrier may be the resistance and scepticism of colleagues, who can view clinical governance as nothing more than 'a mixture of the blindingly obvious (people should lead well and work well in teams) and the unproved (clinical audit)'.[34] Other important obstacles may include: chronic curriculum overload; attitudes which view any curricular content 'beyond' the strictly biomedical as superfluous (and therefore a waste of curricular time); and, of course, the thorny question of how to resource the teaching.

Problem-based learning is mentioned as one approach which 'should in time improve team-working skills'.[16] Its introduction may, in fact, contribute much more, in terms of the acquisition of appropriate skills and attitudes. Although there is controversy concerning some of the benefits claimed by problem-based learning, there are issues pertinent to clinical governance where its approach to teaching and learning could make a significant contribution, not least in the development, enhancement and retention of self-directed learning skills (*see* Box 14.6).[35] Other curricula approaches such as 'guided discovery learning', which combine innovative methods with the best of traditional modes, may also be as effective at promoting self-directed learning.[36]

Three UK medical schools have changed to fully problem-based learning curricula in recent years (Manchester, Liverpool and Glasgow), but several others have adopted problem-based learning in part of their curriculum (e.g. Newcastle, Birmingham, St George's) and this trend is likely to continue.

Box 14.6:   Features of problem-based learning

- *Definition*: 'An educational method characterised by the use of patient problems as a context for students to learn problem-solving skills and acquire knowledge about basic and clinical sciences'.
- *Process*: usually undertaken in small groups that meet two or three times per week and, facilitated by a tutor, follow a series of specific steps in tackling cases and problems.
- *Advantages* (for which there is reasonable evidence): learning is more enjoyable for students and tutors, the learning environment is more stimulating and more humane; self-directed learning skills are enhanced and retained; promotes deep rather than surface learning, greater interaction between students and faculty, and interdepartmental collaboration; students have better interpersonal skills.
- *Advantages* (for which there is weak or conflicting evidence): fosters clinical reasoning and problem-solving skills; promotes retention of knowledge; improves motivation.
- *Disadvantages*: costly in terms of start-up and maintenance costs, including staff time; may be stressful for some students and staff; students acquire less knowledge of basic sciences.

From Finucane *et al.*[33]

Conclusions

This chapter has argued that most of the basic building blocks for learning about clinical governance are already in place in medical undergraduate curricula. Furthermore, a culture is evolving in which *curriculum* governance can provide an analogous framework in which students learn about the basic principles of governance itself.

This process needs to extend to the basic training of all healthcare practitioners and should be seen as a normal part of the curriculum – properly assessed and resourced. Equally, only when clinical governance is seen in action in normal everyday practice will it be taken seriously by all those in training. Failure to do so will have profound implications for the way in which tomorrow's healthcare professionals do their job.

Practical points

- Training future practitioners requires flexibility and vision.
- Undergraduate curricula already address much of the clinical governance agenda.
- Learning about ethics, teamworking, communication with patients and coping with stress is vital for all.
- Curricular governance provides insights for clinical governance.
- The best way to learn is to experience clinical governance in action.

References

1   Calman K (1994) The profession of medicine. *BMJ.* **309**: 1140–3

2   Chastonay P, Brenner E, Peel S and Guilbert J-J (1996) The need for more efficacy and relevance in medical education. *Medical Education.* **30**: 235–8.

3   Donaldson LJ and Muir Gray JA (1998) Clinical governance: a quality duty for health organisations. *Quality in Health Care.* **7**(Suppl 1): S37–44.

4   General Medical Council (1993) *Tomorrow's Doctors. Recommendations on Undergraduate Medical Education.* GMC, London.

5   General Medical Council (1995) *Good Medical Practice.* GMC, London.

6   http://www.ukcc.org.uk

7   Morrison J and Buckley G (1999) Clinical governance – implications for medical education. *Medical Education.* **33**: 162–4.

8   Baker R, Lakhani M, Fraser R and Cheater F (1999) A model for clinical governance in primary care groups. *BMJ.* **318**: 779–80.

9   Morrison JM and Sullivan FM (1997) Audit in general practice: educating medical students. *Medical Education.* **31**: 128–31.

10   Howe AC and Purkiss V (1998) Resourcing innovative teaching of audit – models, methods and MAAGs. *Medical Education.* **32**: 607–12.

11   Evidence-Based Medicine Working Group (1992) Evidence-based medicine. A new approach to teaching the practice of medicine. *JAMA.* **268**: 2420–5.

12   Purves I (1995) *Integrating Medical Informatics into the Medical Undergraduate Curriculum. A Theoretical Overview using Newcastle University as a Template.* Sowerby Unit for Primary Care Informatics, Newcastle.

13   Hope T, Fulford KWM and Yates A (1996) *The Oxford Practice Skills Course.* Oxford University Press, Oxford.

14   Consensus statement by teachers of medical ethics and law in UK medical schools (1998) Teaching medical ethics and law within medical education: a model for the UK core curriculum. *Journal of Medical Ethics.* **24**: 188–92.

15   Coles C (1997) How students learn: the process of learning. In: B Jolly, L Rees (eds) *Medical Education in the Millennium.* Oxford Medical Publications, Oxford, pp 65–7.

16   Scally G and Donaldson LJ (1998) Clinical governance and the drive for quality improvement in the new NHS in England. *BMJ.* **317**: 61–5.

17   Barr H and Waterton S (1996) Summary of a CAIPE survey: interprofessional education in health and social care in the United Kingdom. *Journal of Interprofessional Care.* **10**: 297–303.

18   Boaden N and Bligh J (1999) *Community-Based Medical Education.* Arnold, London.

19   Carpenter J (1995) Doctors and nurses: stereotypes and stereotype change in interprofessional education. *Journal of Interprofessional Care.* **9**: 151–61.

20   British Medical Association (1995) *Core Values for the Medical Profession in the 21st Century: conference report.* BMA, London.

21 Webb E, Ashton H, Kelly P and Kamali F (1998) An update on British medical students' lifestyles. *Medical Education*. **32**: 325–31.

22 Richardson G and Maltby H (1995) Reflection on practice: enhancing student learning. *Journal of Advanced Nursing*. **22**: 235–42.

23 Novack DH, Suchman AL, Clark W, Epstein RM, Najberg E and Kaplan C (1997) Calibrating the physician. Personal awareness and effective patient care. *JAMA*. **278**: 502–9.

24 Elton L (1997) Staff development and the quality of teaching. In: B Jolly and L Rees (eds) *Medical Education in the Millennium*. Oxford Medical Publication, Oxford, pp 199–204.

25 Wilkes M and Bligh J (1999) Evaluating educational interventions. *BMJ*. **318**: 1269–72.

26 Prince CJAH and Visser K (1997) The student as quality controller. In: AJJA Scherpbier, CPM van der Vleuten, JJ Rethans and AFW van der Steed (eds) *Advances in Medical Education*. Kluwer Academic Publishers, Dordrecht, pp 15–18.

27 Visser K, Prince CJ, Scherpbier AJ *et al.* (1998) Student participation in educational management and organisation. *Medical Teacher*. **20**: 451–54.

28 http://www.asme.org.uk/curriculum/liver.htm

29 Stewart M, Belle Brown J, Wayne Weston W, McWhinney IR, McWilliam CL and Freeman TR (1995) *Patient-centred Medicine. Transforming the Clinical Method*. Sage Publications, Thousand Oaks, CA.

30 Jackson P (1996) The student's world. *The Elementary School Journal*. **66**(7): 353.

31 Seabrook M, Lempp H and Woodfield S (1998) *Extending Community Involvement in Medical Education: a guide*. King's Undergraduate Medical Education in the Community, London.

32 Oswald NTA (1996) Doctors for the 21st century: the contribution primary medical care could make. *Education for Health*. **9**: 37–44.

33 Gale R and Grant J (1990) *Managing Change in a Medical Context: guidelines for action*. The Joint Centre, London.

34 Goodman N (1998) Clinical governance. *BMJ*. **317**: 1725–7.

35 Finucane PM, Johnson SM and Prideaux DJ (1998) Problem-based learning; its rationale and efficacy. *Medical Journal of Australia*. **168**: 445–8.

36 Spencer JA and Jordan RK (1999) Learner centred approaches in medical education. *BMJ*. **318**: 1280–3.

CHAPTER 15

The end of certainty: professionalism re-visited

Jamie Harrison and Robert Innes

All professions are conspiracies against the laity

George Bernard Shaw

> This chapter explores what it means to be health service professionals for today. After all, what is 'health'? And, how, against a background of rising expectations of healthcare, can clinical governance help to define and enhance the future 'bargain' between the practitioner and the patient?

The right to health

According to the World Health Organisation (WHO), the possession of health is a basic human right.[1] Since the 18th century, the question of whether individuals have a 'right to health' has been keenly debated. Indeed, the French Revolutionary 'Health Committee of the National Constituent Assembly' formally supported the idea that health was a natural right to which all citizens were entitled, asserting that if the role of government was to protect natural rights, then public health was a duty of the state. More recently, the WHO itself has taken up the campaign of 'Health for all by the year 2000'.

Yet governments struggle to make sense of health planning and the provision of health services. The power of consumerist electorates has driven them into defensive mode, as they try to keep up with burgeoning expectations. Thomas Osborne summarises the position:

> *From the idea that it is the duty of a government to secure the well-being of the population, it is not such a large step – and a nice instance, besides, of the strategic 'reversibility' of power relations – to the parallel idea that it is a right of the population to be provided with health and well-being.*[2]

To be required to guarantee health and wellbeing to the population is, of course, quite different from having to provide access to essential healthcare to individuals and families.[3] Equally, using the language of rights may be mistaken. Rights are, in principle, capable of being asserted against some body (individual or corporate). But individuals are primarily responsible for their own health. And how can a person assert a right against themselves?

Defining health

> *Health is one of a number of words which are constantly in use which are so rich in meaning that they cannot be explained fully without involving controversy.*[4]

The definition of 'health' itself is difficult. As soon as it comes into view, health escapes over the horizon, to reposition itself. This remains a nightmare for policy makers, as much as for practitioners. What was accepted as a reasonable state of health a few years ago – the odd back pain, an occasional cold and intermittent bouts of indigestion – may now be seen as deeply unhealthy. Even one (however tragic) death from meningitis is apparently unacceptable. Being healthy seems increasingly unattainable. Osborne goes on to quote philosopher Georges Canguilhem's provocative point:

> *Health is essentially a negative state rather than a positive one; when one is healthy one is oblivious of the issue of health or ill-health as a problem.*[2]

For Canguilhem, health is something we cannot know positively; or at least we can only know it, so to speak, in its absence. This makes defining health even harder.

Some definitions of health describe an ideal state of being, an *end* in itself, which all might attain (i.e. perfect health). Others delineate health pragmatically, as the *means* which enables people to live a proper life (i.e. the vehicle to self-realisation). The WHO definition of health as *'a state of complete physical, mental and social well-being, not merely the absence of disease and handicap'*[1] is an example of the former approach. Idealised definitions, whilst laying down markers for action, place the proffered ideal state outside the realm of real persons.

The risk of such universal, perfectionist approaches is that they undermine the efforts of those who set out on the quest to establish health. Who would not give up as the impossibility of the task became apparent? And what patient could possibly experience such a Utopian state for any length of time? The claims made by ordinary citizens who might embrace such a definition simply could not be fulfilled by any government or health service. The result could be that the power of medicine is overestimated, and that permanently excessive demands are put on doctors.

The second approach is illustrated by the writings of German theologian Jürgen Moltmann. For Moltmann, health is *'the strength to be human'*.[5] Here, the intention is to portray health as the means by which human beings achieve their full potential. Obstacles to health, whether they be biological, environmental, societal, familial or personal, must be faced and overcome. 'Strength' is not to be equated with strong muscles or performance on a treadmill test. Rather, it is that person-specific quality, utilised by individuals, as they work towards living a fulfilled life. David Seedhouse values how the humanist Katherine Mansfield puts it:

> By health I mean the power to live a full adult, living, breathing, life ... I want to be all that I am capable of becoming.

Seedhouse goes on to talk of health as an essentially enabling quality. It is about providing *'appropriate foundations for achieving potential.'*[4]

Rights, responsibilities and clinical governance

To be fair to the World Health Organisation, the Alma-Ata Declaration speaks of both rights and responsibilities:

> For their part, the people will learn to identify their real health needs and to become involved in and promote community action for health. Thus, society will come to realise that health is not only the right of all but also the **responsibility** of all, and the members of the health professionals, too, will find their proper role.[3]

Yet, encouraging individuals to assume the primary responsibility for their own health is notoriously difficult. Alastair Campbell notes the critique of René Dubos:

> To ward off disease or recover health, man as a rule finds it easier to depend on healers than to attempt the more difficult task of living wisely.[6]

The challenge for clinical governance is clear. How do you set about improving service quality, and safeguarding high standards, without at the same time encouraging a culture of dependency and false expectation amongst patients? (This has been a criticism of government charters.) For to live out one's full humanity, with all its problems, will involve negotiation between what is possible, what is desirable and what should be left well alone.

Promising an excellent service could set the ideal so high that it does no one any favours – confusing the offer of health with that of happiness. One of our most urgent requirements is to find a more adequate definition of health, whilst at the same time making much clearer in the public imagination the strictly limited role that medical intervention has in securing health.

This is a difficult theme, as it contradicts the popular model of modern medicine, where every promise can be fulfilled, even, perhaps, making people happy.[7] The perceived shortcomings of technological medicine (for all its successes) opens the question of who is to blame when things go wrong or, at least, do not follow the perfect plan. For in an individualistic, post-modern world someone or something must be to blame. As Campbell writes:

> the practice of medicine is all too easily destroyed by the inappropriate expectations of patients and by the false pretensions of doctors.[6]

Litigation

We are all conscious of the need to address malpractice and underperformance. Yet society must ask itself at what point pursuing practitioners to maximise their clinical performance becomes counter-productive. For instance, it has become increasingly hard to find an obstetrician in some parts of the USA, such has become the cost of indemnity insurance and the risk of litigation. The desire for a perfect baby has its difficulties.

> American attitudes have exacerbated the situation. There, consumerism dominates medicine. With the right treatment, doctor and hospital, nothing need ever kill you. If anything goes wrong you – or your relatives – can always sue.[8]

So what does constitute a reasonable or adequate or acceptable level of clinical service? If only the best is good enough, and clinical governance expects high standards to be safeguarded and quality continuously improved, then the highest performing unit for every sub-speciality would need to be identified, its level of performance noted.

But would all other, similar, but less effective units be required to close? One criticism of the Bristol cardiac surgery unit was that the performance of the surgeons was not up to that of, say, those at Great Ormond Street. Should all cases, then, go to the national centre (in this case in London) where the team has the exclusive expertise?

An increase in litigation may reflect a loss of trust in the promises that modernity (especially modern, scientific medicine) seemed to be making. At the same time, Utopian notions of health involve a heightened desire for the risk-free (perfect) existence. Yet, most people's experience is of a progressive awareness of their own mortality. This goes with the fragmentation of the support structures of life. How, then, to hold on to the wonder which is life itself?

> From one perspective indeed a human life is not of much significance – birth, growth, death in the space of a few years. Yet that being is capable of loving and being loved, and in consequence is of great value.[9]

The practitioner's task does not come to an end when the resources of curative medical science are exhausted. He or she is required to exercise the love and care of a friend, being with, and affirming, the one who is dying.[10]

From regulation to risk society

Allied to this shift in sensibility from trust towards litigation has been the move from a regulated society to one characterised by risk.[11] The old nationalised bureaucracies (public utilities, rail and air travel, etc.) have been privatised. Deregulation has been the trend of the last decade. With this deregulation comes uncertainty, flexibility and risk. Will it work? Who will pick up the pieces if it doesn't? Will the 'nanny state' still be there when we need her?

At the same time, the general public has been exposed to a catalogue of looming disasters, from 'decimation' through HIV/AIDS, new variant CJD and 'flesh-eating bugs' to the sudden, overwhelming threat of meningitis. It is not, therefore, surprising that there is disquiet when people hear of doctors failing in the simpler tasks. Governments worry too:

> *A risk society, based on deregulation and devolution, often requires more subtle and systematic forms of control. For example, the state is forced to create regulatory systems of quality control where public utilities have been privatized.*[12]

The formation of primary care groups opens up the spectre of small, flexible, budget-limited healthcare organisations being required to manage the risks present in their local health domains. What then is the role of the professional in such an organisation, which is increasingly being asked to provide a uniformly high standard of service to the general public? And at a time when the medical profession is itself under severe scrutiny from itself, the public and the media alike.[13,14]

The nature of professionalism

Much has been made recently of the moves towards revalidation by the GMC and the potential powers of the Commission for Health Improvement. How much should the professional, especially those in a publicly funded service, be directly supervised and how much left to his or her own monitoring of performance? How much should peers be encouraged to participate in performance review? Will they be objective or will they collude? What also of patients – the 'consumers' of the 'product'? In what ways should they be involved?

For at a fundamental level, an understanding of what goes on between the patient and the doctor or nurse must be shared and agreed. What is this so-called 'bargain' that must be struck between them? How does this relationship differ from that between customer and salesman, or master and servant? Does it matter whether you are in a public or a private organisation? Are health professionals contracted or covenanted to their patients? In what ways do patients behave as good citizens, with virtues and responsibilities? (*see* Box 15.1).

Box 15.1:   Characteristics of citizens and professionals

The Good Citizen
Expert on own body
Expects good care
Responsible
Realistic
Informed
Experiences whole of life
Accepts a team response
Assumes effective regulation
Respects professionalism

The Professional
Humble
Consistently competent
Responsive
Accessible
Keeps up-to-date
Flexible
Teamworker
Self-regulating
Follows code of conduct

Partnership between professional carers and those for whom they care points one way forward. Yet all partnerships risk exploitative relationships, either in terms of unequal power relations, or in terms of expecting too much of the other. As one young doctor comments – *doctors offered everything on the basis that patients would not ask too much.*[15] For too long, doctors, in particular, seemed to hold the upper hand. Are patients now asking for more? Ken Jarrold puts this issue into stark relief:

> *Although we often only pay lip service to their existence, patients and carers are at the heart of the NHS. Although events at Bristol and in many other places may give the impression that the NHS exists for the benefit of professional staff – it does not. The NHS exists for patients and carers.*[16]

A culture of professionalism and partnership must be fostered. Without it, patients really do just become objects of the financial machine, viewed either as 'consumers' or as 'sources of income'. But, in an increasingly suspicious and fragmented age, how can such a culture be sustained? (Box 15.2).

Box 15.2:   Attitudes affecting the citizen–professional relationship

Negatively
criticism
contempt
defensiveness
withdrawal

Positively
encouragement
openness
respect
engagement

Power, transparency and interpretation

If, indeed, patients are to work in partnership with their professional carers, then transparency and honesty on both sides are necessary. In an increasingly complex technological age, where information overloads the consultation and both doctor and patient can become more and more bewildered by facts and opinions, shared understandings take on a new significance.

Ian Purves writes of doctor–patient interactions in which 'the computer needs to become the third member in the triadic relationship of the consultation.'[17] The computer offers up 'information' which the doctor seeks to integrate into the patient's story. Informed, shared decision-making follows, as narrative and objective clinical data are synthesised. This 'hermeneutical'[18] process can then lead to a writing of the story for the future, after the consultation. In this way, rights are replaced by partnerships, or covenanted relationships, and both patient and health professional are seen as bearing equal responsibility in the attempt to produce, or maintain, an acceptable state of health and wellbeing.

Hermeneutics and healing

So questions emerge for both patients and practitioners. Is medicine a science or an art? A technique or a practice? Our contemporary culture emphasises the predominance of science, the medical world itself according most prestige to the technical work of specialists, rather than to the personal role of generalists.

But a moment's reflection makes it obvious that medicine is not pure science. William Osler called medicine '*a science of uncertainty and an art of probability.*'[19] Illness is a subjective state. As such, it is not exactly reducible to objective measurements. A patient walks in the surgery and the doctor asks 'How are you?' The question cannot be answered in the language of pure science. Or, at least, anyone who tries to answer it in this way has misunderstood the way in which the language works.

The healer's art begins with listening to the patient's self-description, with sufficient attentiveness and warmth, to gain the patient's trust for the whole story. Here begins the work of clinical wisdom, for what follows is the beginning of an interpretation about what is going on in the patient's life and body. Without this initial way into the patient's story, all that should follow – the early judgement, working diagnosis and subsequent prognosis – is lost.

Obviously, science has a vital place, but scientific reasoning does not, of itself, lead to action. The science must be integrated into the biography of the particular patient (the narrative) and vice versa, so that deductive and practical reasoning lead to wise action – what Ian Purves has called '*the art and the science of the art of medicine.*'[17]

Clinical governance and the bargain with patients

The peculiar mix of art and science appears paradoxical. Patients on the one hand demand rationality, but on the other hand hate the idea that they can be rationalised (and, in addition, fear that services to them may be rationed). No one wants to be thought of as a mere machine.

Successful medicine entails the restoration of wholeness or, at least, fosters the patient's own strength to be human – cooperating with the body's own natural healing processes, with minimal interference. Gadamer gives the illustration of tree-cutting with a two-handed saw – two persons working together harmoniously. But if one person applies too much force, the blade jams.[20]

This analogy, of the two-handed saw, also applies to the bargain between patients and practitioners. For clinical governance to work effectively, this relationship must be both transparent and cooperative in nature. It is no longer permissible to claim a professional monopoly of power in the healing process. Patients have the right to equal partnership. NHS organisations are accountable to them. They deserve high standards, indeed, excellence of care, as the governance definition puts it.

Yet patients already recognise that doctors and nurses are under severe pressure at work. They do not wish to see this pressure increase, and are willing to share the burdens of decision-making in the health service. They respect those who care for them (*see* Box 15.3).

Box 15.3:   Good citizen–professional interactions

- manifest consistent technical soundness
- engage the whole human experience
- recognise the citizen as a person with unique identity and responsibility
- use resources appropriately
- lead to mutually acceptable outcomes
- help to improve the health of individuals and populations
- are realistic and affirming
- share responsibility and decision-making

Equally, workers in primary care need to demonstrate their respect for patients, by listening and allowing them the space, and the capacity, to offer an opinion and to criticise the professional viewpoint as and when appropriate.

Gadamer suggests that, to preserve a proper attitude to one's own authority as a professional, one needs to be free to make mistakes on occasions, and to be able to recognise the fact.[20] Appropriate structures of governance must be designed so that they do not inhibit the healer's ability to admit mistakes inwardly, to colleagues or to patients, whilst at the same time not putting the public at excessive risk. A no-blame, supportive culture, with mutuality, should be the goal. Without such a culture, governance becomes something to fear and its presence seen as an unwarranted imposition. That benefits neither practitioners nor patients.

Practical points

- Idealised definitions of health lead to unrealistic expectations.
- These are fuelled by the pretensions of scientific medicine.
- The challenge for clinical governance is how to improve service quality without encouraging dependency and false expectations among patients.
- Partnership between professionals and citizens points a way forward.
- Patients rightly expect high standards, but also recognise practitioners are under severe pressure.
- As citizens they are willing to share decision-making in the health service.

References

1   WHO (1948) *The Constitution of the World Health Organisation.* WHO, Geneva.

2   Osborne T (1997) Of health and statecraft. In: A Petersen and R Bunton (eds) *Foucault, Health and Medicine.* Routledge, London.

3   WHO and UNICEF (1978) *Primary Health Care (The Alma-Ata Report).* Geneva/New York.

4   Seedhouse D (1986) *Health: the foundation for achievement.* Wiley, Chichester.

5   Moltmann J (1985) *God in Creation. An Ecological Doctrine of Creation.* SCM Press, London.

6   Campbell AV (1984) *Moderated Love: a theology of professional care.* SPCK, London.

7   Harrison J (1998) Post-modern influences. In: J Harrison and T van Zwanenberg (eds) *GP Tomorrow.* Radcliffe Medical Press, Oxford.

8   Coward R (1999) Go to bed. *The Guardian.* 9 January.

9   Smith B (1998) *The Silence of Divine Love.* Darton, Longman and Todd, London.

10 Illich I (1995) Death undefeated. From medicine to medicalization to systematization. *BMJ.* **311**: 1652–3.

11 Beck U (1992) *Risk Society. Towards a New Modernity.* Sage, London.

12 Turner BS (1997) From governmentality to risk. In: A Petersen and R Bunton (eds) *Foucault, Health and Medicine.* Routledge, London.

13 Lough M (1999) *Paper on clinical governance presented at the UK Conference of Regional Advisors in General Practice.* RCGP, London, 28 January.

14   Harrison J (1996) Is this what we really want? *BMJ*. **313**: 1643; see also Harrison J and Innes R (1997) *Medical Vocation and Generation X*. Grove Books, Cambridge.

15   Vaughan C and Higgs R (1995) Doctors and commitment. Nice work – shame about the job. *BMJ*. **311**: 1654–5.

16   Jarrold K (1998) *Servants and leaders: leadership in the NHS*. University of York lecture, 30 July.

17   Purves I (1998) The changing consultation. In: J Harrison and T van Zwanenberg (eds) *GP Tomorrow*. Radcliffe Medical Press, Oxford.

18   Hermeneutics is the study of interpretation. The hermeneutical process is the task of the doctor or nurse in interpreting the patient's story in the light of both that narrative and the scientific evidence available.

19   Pellegrino ED and Thomasma DC (1981) *A Philosophical Basis of Medical Practice: toward a philosophy and ethic of the healing professions*. Oxford University Press, Oxford.

20   Gadamer H-G (1996) *The Enigma of Health: the art of healing in a scientific age*. Blackwells, Oxford.

CHAPTER SIXTEEN

Implementing clinical governance

Jamie Harrison and Tim van Zwanenberg

For every difficult and complicated question, there is an answer that is simple, easily understood and wrong.

HL Mencken

Primary care faces many challenges at the beginning of a new millennium. This concluding chapter examines the broad issues to be faced as the era of clinical governance dawns.

Clinical governance in action

So what, then, is clinical governance? The complementary themes within this book, taken together, seek to paint a picture in which clinical governance is portrayed as the means whereby the issue of quality in primary care can be addressed. Yet each individual and team within primary care may receive the light slanted across the canvas differently, and so perceive the image with slight alterations in comparison with their neighbours.

Or, to take the analogy of the stained glass window, the message of the whole set of panes can change with the quality and quantity of light, the position of the observer and their willingness to engage with the process of looking. Education may be needed in how to interpret the contents of the image, and simplistic answers to what it 'means' will need to be challenged.

For, undoubtedly, some claiming expertise will appear, offering short-cuts and comfortable options, on the road to clinical governance. Yet common sense dictates that to achieve the proper implementation of clinical governance will take time and effort. Indeed, the government itself has a 10-year timetable for improving the quality of clinical care.

But there are decisions to be taken, and dilemmas to be resolved, in relation to the clinical governance agenda in the here and now. How will primary care begin to measure up to such challenges? And what are the risks it will run, should it choose to avoid answering the questions that are being posed?

Communication or confusion?

One significant question for the culture of primary care relates to its willingness to improve communications – both internally and with outsiders. Sadly, patients often fit into the latter grouping. Regular communication within teams, proper consultation mechanisms and effective ways of passing on information, lead to a greater ownership of the service by all, more efficiency, less confusion, and, hopefully, better clinical care and job satisfaction.

Humility or hubris?

Both these words are misunderstood. Humility is misrepresented as weakness; hubris as confident leadership. True humility allows others to make their contribution, values participation in decision-making, and is willing to learn. Hubris is arrogant power-seeking, presumption of unearned authority. The doctor no longer automatically knows what is best for the patient – the same can be said for any single health professional in primary care.

Courage or complacency?

It is easiest to do nothing, especially in the face of major change. Inertia soon gains the upper hand. There must, of course, be proper discussion about how to respond to change, with leadership, clarity and time for reflection. The speed of response needs to be measured, with careful planning and realism. But there may also need to be courage, living out a belief in what is possible, achievable and necessary.

Inclusivity or isolationism?

Should all be included? Does the definition of 'all' need some thought? It is so easy to leave someone out, intentionally or unintentionally. With new primary care team, primary care group and primary care trust structures in place, work will be needed if all are to feel included. Equally, limited horizons can make for delusions of success and false ideas that all is well. We need each other. Strength comes from sharing and seeing the bigger picture, not from being isolated.

Partnership or protectionism?

It is traditional to close ranks when the pressure arrives. Professional self-interest is a powerful force, not only in primary care. Yet the clinical governance agenda calls for the rejection of historical protectionism, replacing it with openness and transparency. Patients, politicians and professionals share many common values and beliefs. Decisions about issues of life and death, the rationing of services and our common future would seem more helpfully made together rather than apart.

Conclusion

Clinical governance offers to all in primary care the opportunity to celebrate success, as much as to look to improve. It is all too easy to forget that most things are done well, that society values primary care's efforts highly, and that each new generation of doctors, nurses and managers builds on the contribution of its predecessors.

Yet, equally, there is room to make improvements across the board. Using creativity and simplicity, the new clinical governance agenda can be tackled effectively and systematically. It is, of course, an agenda which is both exciting and not a little daunting.

Index